HERBAL REMEDIES

A practical guide to herbs and their healing properties

NICOLA PETERSON

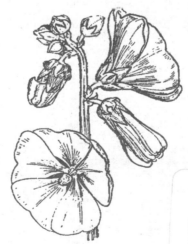

BLITZ EDITIONS

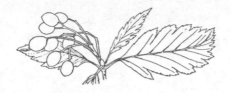

Published by Blitz Editions
an imprint of Bookmart Ltd
Registered Number 2372865
Trading as Bookmart Ltd
Desford Road
Enderby
Leicester LE9 5AD

This book created by Amazon Publishing Ltd, Middlesex
Editor: Diana Russell
Design: Wilson Design Associates
Cover photography: Andrew Kolesnikow
Printed and bound in Great Britain by
BPC Hazell Books Ltd
A member of
The British Printing Company Ltd

ISBN 1-85605-330-X

SAFETY NOTE
Throughout the book *asterisks refer to important safety
information placed in boxes below the marked text. Please read these notes carefully.

AUTHOR'S NOTE
All recommendations contained in this book are believed by the author to be effective if
properly administered and if the correct, good-quality herbs are used. However, the author has
no control over the herbs used by others or the manner in which they are used, and the author
cannot guarantee the effectiveness of their use or be held in any way liable.

If you are in any doubt about the nature of your illness, the author strongly recommends
you seek the advice of your doctor or other qualified medical practitioner.

CONTENTS

INTRODUCTION

My nine-year-old son says I am plant-mad. I suppose as I have gone from wanting to be a florist at fourteen years of age to working as a gardener in my twenties and qualifying as a herbal practitioner at the age of twenty-eight there could be something in this. All I can say is that the more I have learnt and experienced about the work, the more fascinating and rewarding I have found it. The other great privilege of working as a practitioner is the contact I have with my patients. Working together with so many over the last dozen or so years, using a system of medicine that acknowledges the innate self-healing actions of the body has taught me a great deal about life in general that I am very aware of and grateful for.

I hope this book will pass on some of my knowledge and enthusiasm for the use of plants. It is not inherently a mystifying or obscure subject - in fact a few generations ago traditional family knowledge about helpful plants was the first step in the treatment of minor illnesses. I hope to restore some of that knowledge to people who are interested in finding a safe and effective alternative to over-the-counter pharmaceuticals in use for such illnesses.

A final word, however. Although herbs can bring great benefits, not all are suitable for all conditions. For example, to err on the side of caution you should avoid certain herbs in pregnancy. Throughout this book, safety information and other important notes are presented in boxes, with passages in the text marked with an *asterisk if they relate directly to information in a box on the page.

CHAPTER 1

WHAT IS HERBAL MEDICINE?

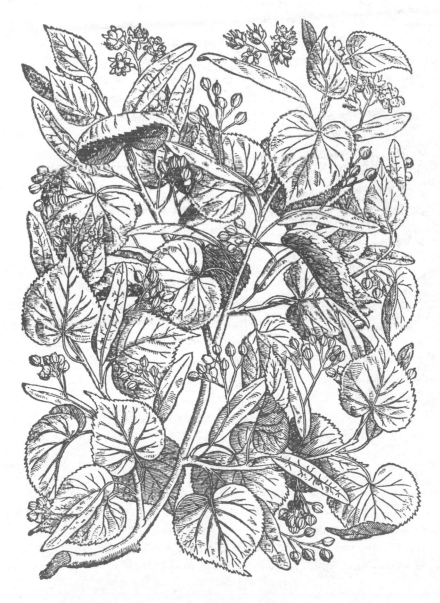

By the time the human race evolved about 150,000 years ago, land plants had already been in existence for 400 million years. Great diversity had developed, yielding an enormous range of naturally produced chemical constituents. As civilization developed, people came to know which plants were good to eat and which were good to help against disease. Herbal medicine is the skill of using one's knowledge of the effects of plants to benefit the health of a person.

This was the only type of medicine available to people for thousands of years in the past. It is still the most easily-available medicine in many parts of the world today.

In the West the best phrase to describe the herbalist's approach is 'the whole plant for the whole person'. Why the whole plant? Because the enormous range and subtle combination of constituents in a plant will give it a unique action that cannot be duplicated by anything synthetic. Why the whole person? Because herbalists respect every patient as a unique individual and look for the cause of a disease rather than just examining the symptoms. Also, instead of giving a standardized preparation a herbalist will usually make a unique combination of remedies to fit the needs of the individual patient as closely as possible.

HOW DOES IT WORK?

It is not easy to draw a dividing line between herbal medicine and nutrition. Many plants we eat as foods have quite strong actions on the body and the amount that can safely be eaten will vary from person to person - for instance, spicy foods cause some people drastic stomach problems while others can eat curries every day. The hot drinks we are all familiar with, namely tea and coffee, should definitely be classed as herbs rather than foods and can have very strong effects if taken in excess. So

everybody is affected in certain ways by the
plants that form part of their diets, apart from
the most straightforward questions of nutrition.

Most people in the world eat a range of plants
every day. Our bodies are used to consuming
them, absorbing what is beneficial to us and
getting rid of the waste products. Given that there
are millions of biochemical processes going on
in our bodies all the time and that there are
millions of chemical substances in plants, it isn't
too surprising that many plants have constituents
that do have an effect on how our bodies work.
Not all plants have beneficial effects - just
because it is natural doesn't necessarily mean it is safe.
Some plants are known to be poisonous, and
indeed we have to warn children against being
tempted to eat berries and leaves from the wild. We
know for example that digoxin, a substance found in *foxglove leaves,
helps to strengthen the beating of the heart but that it can be very
dangerous at the wrong dose.

C A U T I O N

Foxglove is not a herb that should be taken by the layperson.
Senna is best avoided during pregnancy and should only be taken under
medical supervision.

Many herbs work by stimulating functions of the body that may not be
working effectively enough by themselves; for instance, *senna pods are
about the best-known herbal remedy because they correct that most
widespread problem of underactive function, constipation. Some remedies
help to calm down overactive functioning, such as those that have a
relaxing and calming action on the nervous system.

This explanation is based on the prevailing scientific view of medicine we have in the West. Cultures in other parts of the world may have very different ways of looking at life, and consequently very different ways of understanding how herbal remedies work. It is certainly true that in my work as a practitioner over the last twelve years I have learnt that not everything involving people's health can be explained scientifically, and that it is more realistic to admit what we don't know. The 'tender loving care' factor can never be discounted in any type of medicine, and relationships are important. Herbal practitioners will have respect for their patients and the remedies, and will acknowledge that the outcome of the treatment may depend as much on what the patient is prepared to do to help her or himself as on whatever medicine is prescribed.

WHAT CAN HERBAL REMEDIES DO FOR YOU?

Because the herbs that are featured in this book are all quite safe to use when the advice given is followed, they are ideal for treating a wide range of minor domestic health problems. In addition, some of them can help reduce the risk of succumbing to infections like coughs and colds, and can be taken as 'insurance' by people who are susceptible to these problems. Some can be taken regularly as aids to the normal functioning of various parts of the body that might be temporarily or permanently under par, such as the digestion. Because these remedies are so well tolerated, they can be thought of almost as part of a person's normal diet rather than as a specifically medical item. Even for those in good health, herbal teas can make pleasant and refreshing drinks free from the problems of caffeine-stimulation that tea and coffee cause.

It would be misleading for me to suggest that herbal medicine is always completely successful – I don't know of any system of medicine that could be so. What I do know from personal experience, however, is that there is almost always something that is worth trying. Any change that contributes to a healthier way of life will pay off sooner or later, and you may find a new interest in gardening or botany along the way!

Chapter 4 of this book contains much more information about the substances we now know that herbs contain, and about the actions they have on the body. Chapter 6 provides an alphabetical guide to the herbs and their uses, while Chapter 7 suggests which remedies to use for which problems, with a brief explanation of the way they work. By reading these chapters you will understand much more about the approach to illness that herbalists adopt, and how remedies are chosen for specific health problems.

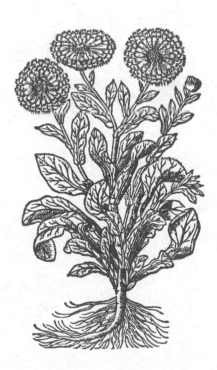

A BRIEF HISTORY OF HERBAL MEDICINE

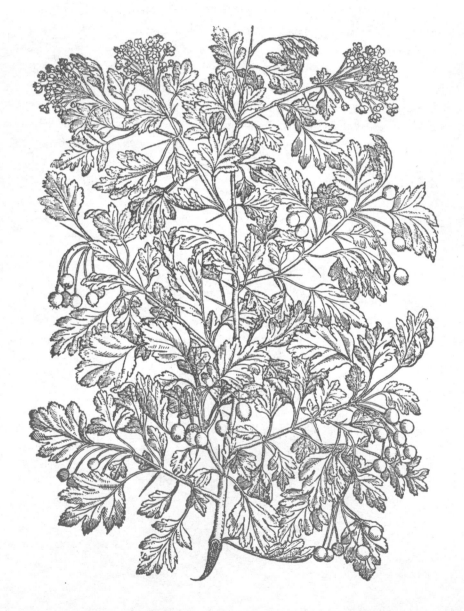

Although we have no direct way of knowing about the importance of medicinal plants to early humans, we can make informed theories based on several lines of evidence. The two most relevant come from archaeology and anthropology: the study of modern-day tribes that have been isolated from outside influences until very recently. Archaeological remains have shown that various plants were included in burial rituals. Some of these have been in good enough condition to be identified, and have turned out to be plants that are still used in folk medicine where they are available. In ancient cultures such as those of China and Egypt, where written records were left, accounts of the use of herbal medicines have been found.

An idea of the place of herbs in the earliest societies is probably best suggested by their use in current isolated tribes. Here, any plant that is of value to human life, whether nutritionally, medicinally or economically (for building shelters, making ropes, nets, etc.), is highly valued. In ancient societies, certain remedies would have been well known to all members of the community and used for minor problems. There was probably a separate body of knowledge, more detailed, known only to the initiated few, whom other members of the group would have called on for help if an illness was too difficult for them to deal with. These 'specialists' might also have had some religious role in the group, and their knowledge was passed on only to their successors.

At an early stage of civilization it would have been very important to make good observations of the efficacy (or not) of treatments, to develop the knowledge and skills of the initiates. Trial and error would have been the first type of scientific method. There must have been many errors, but over the generations a useful body of knowledge about medicinal plants was built up: getting it right was literally vital.

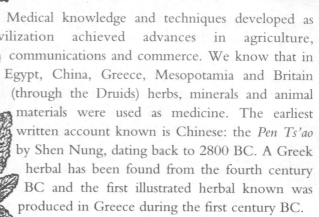

Medical knowledge and techniques developed as civilization achieved advances in agriculture, communications and commerce. We know that in Egypt, China, Greece, Mesopotamia and Britain (through the Druids) herbs, minerals and animal materials were used as medicine. The earliest written account known is Chinese: the *Pen Ts'ao* by Shen Nung, dating back to 2800 BC. A Greek herbal has been found from the fourth century BC and the first illustrated herbal known was produced in Greece during the first century BC.

The Roman empire drew together in learning and commerce the whole of the Mediterranean lands, and numbers of valuable plants spread to previously uncolonized areas. Rome looked after the health of its armies well, and Roman doctors took their skills to all parts of the empire. This resulted in a cross-fertilization with the medical knowledge of local cultures. After the dissolution of the Roman empire society became more fragmented, and medicine in Europe came to adhere rigidly to a system developed by a practitioner named Galen in the second century AD. He created a complex system of classifying illnesses and the remedies that were appropriate for their treatment: this was the first time that theories and models rather than direct observation came to hold sway.

This meant the parting of the ways between 'amateur' and professional practitioner. The amateurs, often local people with a family tradition, tended to prescribe relatively simple and easily available medicines based on their own experience of what was effective. Professional practitioners who had been trained in the Galenic classifications tended to favour more complex and exotic prescriptions, and often used more aggressive interventions such as purging and blood-letting.

Britain was comparatively enlightened at this time, as there was a tradition which followed the principles of the great Greek medical thinker, Hippocrates, developed 600 years before Galen. This approach stressed the concept of a healthy lifestyle, and illness was seen in the context of a person's way of life. Good diet, healthy exercise and happiness were regarded as the cornerstones of health, and treatment was geared towards supporting these where possible. This tradition was kept alive for hundreds of years by the Myddfai practitioners (named after the part of Wales where it originated). It was influential in Britain throughout Saxon times, and served the community well until the next great development in medicine arrived.

FROM THE EARLY CHRISTIAN PERIOD TO CULPEPER AND WESLEY

In AD 597 Christianity was introduced into Britain. The monasteries were part of a network of knowledge and culture that spanned the whole of Europe. The monks saw helping the sick as part of their spiritual calling, and every monastery came to have its own infirmary and physic garden. Although not originally trained as the professionals were, monks eventually came to take over the training of doctors because of their efficiency and success in the work. Support for this from Alfred the Great in the late ninth century made England the most medically advanced country in Europe at that time.

Great developments were also being made in the Arab world. Many Greek and Roman texts had been taken to the Middle East and were used as the basis for further study. The initiative for further investigation and development of medicine passed to the Arab world, while Europe became rather conservative, relying more rigidly on what had been devised in previous centuries. As a consequence, great Arab physicians like Avicenna (Ibn Said) at the end of

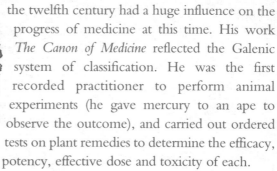

the twelfth century had a huge influence on the progress of medicine at this time. His work *The Canon of Medicine* reflected the Galenic system of classification. He was the first recorded practitioner to perform animal experiments (he gave mercury to an ape to observe the outcome), and carried out ordered tests on plant remedies to determine the efficacy, potency, effective dose and toxicity of each.

European practitioners benefited from these studies. As commerce and the skills of apothecaries grew, more and more remedies became available. The art of preserving and formulating various liquids and ointments developed, and costly exotic remedies, available only through the apothecaries' trade, earned them a good income. Doctors came increasingly to prescribe complex combinations of exotics, possibly thinking that after their long academic training they should come up with something different from that which any countrywoman might have growing in her garden for free. Neither doctors nor apothecaries could make a living by suggesting people should treat themselves with something that was growing in their own gardens!

The superior status of trained doctors was also jeopardized by plagues like the Black Death in the thirteenth century, where the professionals had no more success than the 'amateur' herbalists. As the doctors' treatments included bleeding, purging and the use of toxic substances like mercury and arsenic, this was hardly surprising.

By the time of Henry VII in the early sixteenth century all sorts of medical practitioners, trained and untrained, were flourishing in London. Henry himself had a keen interest in herbal medicine, and most country wives would have known the basics of what their garden plants had to offer. Books on the subject were becoming available with the advent of printing and the increase in reading skills among the people. Great works like that of John Gerard (1545-1607), famous as a master-surgeon and gardener, helped establish an accessible body of knowledge. Some sort of regulation was deemed necessary and several Acts of Parliament were passed, acknowledging the superior status of physicians and ascribing places lower in the hierarchy to surgeons, barber-surgeons and apothecaries.

Unlicensed practitioners – that is simple herbalists – were as a result discriminated against and in some cases prosecution was considered. This brought about a backlash wave of support for the herbalists, including from people in high places, and another Act was passed to protect men and women 'whom God hath endued with the knowledge of nature, kind and operation of certain Herbs, Roots and Waters, and the using and ministring of them ....'. Thus ordinary people who had no profession to protect them had their rights to practise upheld.

While this was going on in the political arena, other changes were taking place in the practical world of science and medicine. Led by the example of the great Swiss-German doctor Paracelsus, alchemy was delving into the secrets of minerals. Laboratory techniques were being developed that enabled the processing of raw materials, whether of plant, animal or mineral origin. Under the influence of Paracelsus, the idea that extracting the active principles of remedies would improve their use became popular. Side-effects were supposed to be avoided with this approach, and therapeutic benefits were thought to be speeded up.

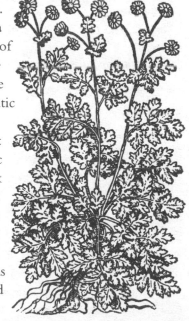

In fact it was the stronger actions that could be immediately seen: dramatic interventions produced gratifyingly quick results such as vomiting and purging. Treatment with whole herbs was less dramatic in comparison and the results took longer to show themselves. The gulf between 'amateur' doctoring in country areas using simple, accessible herbal remedies and the urban use of costly processed medicines

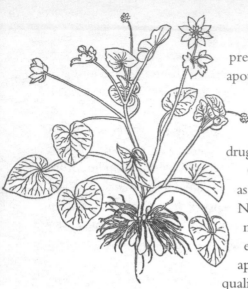

prescribed by doctors and sold by apothecaries continued to grow. It was clear in mid-seventeenth-century society that herbs were the medicine of poor or unfashionable people, and exotics or drugs were for the rich.

One great figure, familiar to most people as the personification of the herbalist, was Nicholas Culpeper (1616-54). He was most unusual in having had a Cambridge education, and then deciding to become apprenticed to an apothecary rather than qualifying as a doctor (which would have been far more financially rewarding). He thundered against the high charges demanded by doctors and the overcomplex prescriptions that brought wealth to the apothecaries, alleging that this type of practice relieved their patients of nothing except money.

In an attempt to reduce their power and status, he translated the standard *Pharmacopoeia* of the time from Latin into English to make it more accessible. Then in due course he wrote the most famous herbal of all: *The English Physician*. This gave clear accounts of all familiar herbal remedies and advised as to which illnesses they would help, without expounding complicated theories. It must have been treasured in thousands of households throughout the country for the value of its straightforward guidance. Throughout his life Culpeper maintained his own practice of herbal medicine, treating the poor of London with simple low-cost remedies. He was followed in the next century by other writers, including the preacher Charles Wesley, who advocated a sensible diet, good hygiene practice, the use of simple herbal remedies and the avoidance of doctors as the best way to stay healthy!

However, by the early nineteenth century even the popular home treatments were becoming more 'mineral-drug' based, and the herbal remedies remaining in use were more likely to be expensive exotics rather than home-grown. Powerful drugs for self-medication could be bought over the counter. Only the poorest people still collected their own (free) fresh herbs. Even throughout this time, however, occasional books about the value of herbal medicine were published. They warned of the risks of drug treatment and exhorted people to keep to the safer, simpler herbs. They were prompted by observations of the damage done by treatments based on calomel (mercury) and laudanum: in fact a study of calomel gave rise to the first published acknowledgment of side-effects in any drug.

DEVELOPMENTS IN THE NEW WORLD

In the seventeenth century the New World had been settled by the first wave of European emigrants. Several plants had already been introduced from the Americas, such as guaiacum (now used for rheumatic problems, at the time of its introduction it was used desperately in the hope of providing a successful treatment against the scourge of syphilis).

Cinchona bark, the original source of the drug quinine, proved to be the first successful treatment for malaria. Interestingly, although it was so successful it was never widely prescribed by professional doctors. They rejected the use of the herb because it was prescribed empirically – that is, because it was observed to help the condition of patients rather than fitting into a theoretical classification. Cinchona was mainly imported by Jesuit priests who had discovered its properties from the native Indians of the New World (one of its alternative names was 'Jesuit bark'). Thus the apothecaries could not monopolize the trade for their own financial advantage and relatively few were interested in stocking it. The Catholic church deserves most of the credit for the success of the fight against malaria in Europe.

Apart from these notable items, most of the potential of American medicinal plants was ignored by the settlers. They preferred to keep to their European ideas and remedies, importing these at great cost from the Old World. There were few trained doctors in America, and as medical schools became established they were dominated by the old European ideas taken to extremes. Blood-letting was considered the supreme treatment, and there are records of up to 2.25 litres (4 pints) at a time being removed. Toxic substances like mercury and antimony were prescribed in larger doses than were ever used in Europe, and the drastic reactions they caused were welcomed as a sign of their activity. Of course, huge numbers of settlers died from these treatments as well as from their original illnesses. Others who survived endured years of painful side-effects. Although the native Americans were acknowledged to be exceptionally healthy and strong people, most Europeanized doctors never considered that 'primitive' Indian medicine might have something to offer the settlers.

Eventually, an empirical type of herbal medicine did develop among the pioneer peoples. This was based purely on the observation of how remedies helped in certain illnesses; its practitioners were non-academic and medically untrained. They were held in great contempt by the orthodox doctors, who brought as much litigation against them as possible. Records suggest that far more of these herbalists' patients recovered from the infectious epidemics that swept the settlements than did those of the doctors. The pioneer of this system at the beginning of the nineteenth century was a farmer called Samuel Thomson. He had seen so much misery inflicted by doctors that he took to treating his family, and then his friends, with herbal remedies that he learnt about from the local herbalist and through his own observations. His system of treatment was developed by experience as more and more people asked for his services.

Thomson's approach was to increase the heat of the body by sitting patients in very hot baths and prescribing remedies like cayenne. Emetics and purges were also used. The basic theory was that this removed the cause of all illness, which was thought to lie in internal 'obstructions' to the circulation of heat around the body. The rest he left to nature.

The treatment was accessible to all because of its low cost, and its use spread through a type of franchise system. It was patented in 1813. A supply of recommended herbs and a handbook explaining their use could be purchased, and the agent thus established became a practitioner. This system became enormously popular, and there were even whole infirmaries dedicated to its practice. Interest in the use of native plants was growing, and several North American herbals were published around this time. The skill of the native people was at last being acknowledged, and their naturopathic techniques such as the use of sweat-lodges became fleetingly popular. These were similar in principle to our modern saunas, with the addition of the use of herbal remedies: plant materials were placed on the hot stones to evaporate.

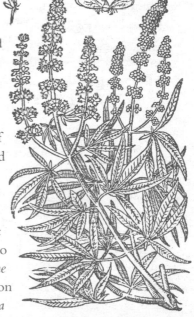

The overall growth in the popularity of herbal medicine constituted a real challenge to the supremacy of the academically trained doctors. A few of the more open-minded among these became interested in herbs themselves, and a movement to reform the excesses of orthodox practice started. Some medical schools even introduced the study of botanical medicine into the curriculum, and several medical schools were founded which were devoted to the teaching of Thomsonian and other herbal or homoeopathic systems. Thomsonian training became more academic and the term 'physiomedicalism' was coined to describe it. Detailed text-books such as *The Philosophy of Physiomedicalism* by J. M. Thurston and *Physio-Medical Therapeutics, Materia Medica*

and Pharmacy by T. J. Lyle (both teachers in physiomedical colleges) became standard works on the subject until well into the twentieth century.

The status of herbal practitioners and homoeopaths was roughly comparable to that of doctors. There were too many poorly trained and often unsuccessful, unpopular doctors graduating from numerous second-rate medical schools. Added to this, the health of Americans, particularly American women, was generally poor – possibly due to the accumulated effects of taking calomel from an early age. This was the lowest point of orthodox medicine in America.

Doctors' fortunes began to change at the end of the nineteenth century when a programme of inspections of all medical schools and unfavourable reports on many of them led to more than half closing over the next thirty years. The resulting improvement in orthodox standards and developments in medical sciences and technology (concerned with chemistry rather than medicinal plants) led to a waning of interest in herbalism. The number of students enrolling at the schools of physiomedicalism was in sharp decline, so that eventually these too were closed.

TOWARDS MODERN PRACTICE

In the UK the practice of herbal medicine was always under threat from orthodox doctors. The fusion of the herbal traditions of Europe and America came about in the middle of the nineteenth century, when an American practitioner named Albert Coffin travelled to France and then England to set up a practice. He became most successful and well established in the north of England, where he publicized his work through lectures and talks for the public. His low-cost remedies (which included both European and American plants) helped hundreds of working-class city-dwellers.

Numerous agents of his, both men and women, set up in practice under his direction in a way similar to the Thomsonian system in America.

Although these practitioners did not have a rigorous academic training they were very aware of the influence of environmental factors on health. Through their experience of life in the cities of northern England, they realized the importance of hygiene. They campaigned for improved sanitation, better food, shorter working hours and better standards of industrial safety for the workers. Their treatment of victims of the mid-nineteenth-century cholera epidemics was easily as successful as that of orthodox doctors. Many of them ran thriving businesses importing herbs from America – a reversal of the situation that had applied 200 years earlier. From its roots in the north the system spread throughout the country. As its success grew it attracted more hostile attention from the medical establishment, and its practitioners were subject to many attempts by doctors to bring prosecutions against them.

Disputes became common among the practitioners – a frequent occurrence in small organizations where beliefs are passionately held – and internal dissent became the greatest destructive force in the end. A public meeting proved to be the scene of the final confrontation between the increasingly autocratic Coffin and his right-hand man, a Devon practitioner named John Skelton. Coffin retired embittered after this, severing his connections with the movement he had led.

Further problems were being caused by the developing pharmaceuticals industry. Active ingredients were being extracted from plants, such as morphine from opium poppies and quinine from cinchona, so that it was no longer considered necessary to use the whole plant as a medicine. Pharmacognosy (the academic study of the identification of plant material) was becoming a normal part of the pharmacist's training.

Traditional herbal medicine was thought to be outdated, and its practitioners were under constant pressure through denunciations by orthodox doctors, court cases, etc. An attempt was made to pass a bill through Parliament to ban unregistered practitioners from working. However, there was still enough support from both the general public and in Parliament to prevent it from becoming law.

The National Association of Medical Herbalists was formed to protect the tradition, and in 1895 it gained the status of a limited company. With a small membership and limited income, it managed to steer a course through all the difficulties to continue the work of herbalists. The north of England was once again its stronghold. With no training school, there were only a few new members coming into practice, and the profession struggled to maintain itself through the early years of the twentieth century.

Matters improved temporarily during the First World War, when medical supplies from Europe were cut off and the public were exhorted to grow whatever medicinal plants they could. Lectures, training courses and information leaflets were produced to meet a huge public demand for knowledge. Garlic was particularly required, as it was used as an antiseptic application to soldiers' wounds (and often the dressing itself was made of sphagnum moss). Numerous herb nurseries were established, but after the war the momentum was lost and many of these went out of business.

Between the wars there was enormous expansion in the orthodox drugs industry, so that by 1939 the demand for herbal medicines was much reduced. A few dedicated people kept the skills alive during this period, notably Mary Grieve and Hilda Leyel. Mary Grieve ran a medicinal herb nursery and organized talks and courses for the public. She will mainly be remembered for writing a range of information pamphlets on herbal remedies that were later collected and published in one volume by Hilda Leyel under the title *A Modern Herbal*. This comprehensive work was a timely addition to the literature on herbal medicine and is still available today. Hilda Leyel was a practitioner herself, founding the Society of Herbalists (now known as the Herb Society) as well as starting Culpeper House to sell herbal preparations to the public. There are branches of this throughout the UK today.

Despite these efforts, by the time of the Second World War there was little widespread interest in herbalism. In the face of hostility from the medical establishment and with no government support, the numbers of practitioners and students were dropping. Finally the National Association, now known as the National Institute of Medical Herbalists (NIMH), suspended its training course completely. A further blow came with the Pharmacy and Medicines Act 1941, which withdrew practitioners' rights to supply their patients with medicine. This aroused far more public reaction than had been anticipated, and the letter of the Act was never enforced. Herbal practice continued, but it must have felt a precarious position to the herbalists to be working outside the law.

The 1940s and 50s saw the lowest ebb of herbalism in Britain. The Institute struggled on, supported by the enormous energy of a few practitioners. Among these was Fred Fletcher Hyde, current President Emeritus of the NIMH. His father before him and later his two sons all became Fellows of the Institute for their services to herbal medicine. He devoted his time to maintaining training and fought for the reinstatement of practitioners' rights. The result of this was the Medicines Act 1968, which represented the culmination of four years' hard campaigning to win recognition. Fred Fletcher Hyde was appointed by a government minister to the Committee on the Review of Medicines, the

Committee on Safety of Medicines (Herbal Remedies Committee) and the Prescription Only Committee (Herbal Remedies) of the Medicines Commission. This was the first time that a herbal practitioner had received such recognition from the government.

If the efforts leading to the Medicines Act 1968 had not been made it is unlikely that the profession would have survived. The government was planning to require herbal medicines to be tested in the same way that orthodox drugs were. This would have been prohibitively expensive for the relatively small manufacturing companies involved, none of whom had the wealth of the drugs companies. It took from 1964 to 1968 to achieve recognition of herbal medicines as having a separate status from that of orthodox drugs.

Several strides forward followed. The Act of 1968 meant that UK herbal practitioners had a degree of official recognition. It prompted the founding of the British Herbal Medicine Association (BHMA), an organization comprising both herbal practitioners and manufacturers. The BHMA then

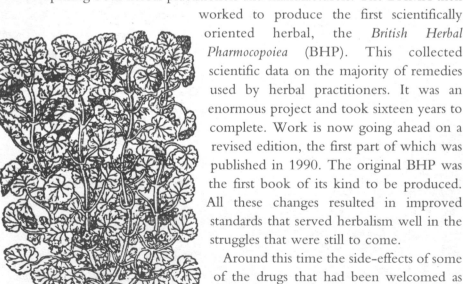

worked to produce the first scientifically oriented herbal, the *British Herbal Pharmocopoiea* (BHP). This collected scientific data on the majority of remedies used by herbal practitioners. It was an enormous project and took sixteen years to complete. Work is now going ahead on a revised edition, the first part of which was published in 1990. The original BHP was the first book of its kind to be produced. All these changes resulted in improved standards that served herbalism well in the struggles that were still to come.

Around this time the side-effects of some of the drugs that had been welcomed as miraculous in the 1950s were starting to appear, and the public were becoming more wary about taking them. Environmental concerns were developing too, while awareness of the dangers of pollution and chemical additives to food also helped to bring about a renewed interest in many forms of 'natural' therapies. By the 1970s the NIMH Education Fund had been set up as a registered charity to raise funds for a school of herbal medicine, which was established by the end of the decade. The number of students completing the training and joining the Institute has risen steadily since then and there are now about 300 members. The most exciting development in training is the BSc course recently started at a university in London. This is a three-year degree course followed by one year's clinical training to gain entry to the NIMH. It is the first time that herbal medicine has gained such academic acceptance.

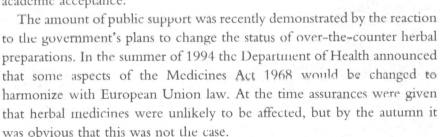

The amount of public support was recently demonstrated by the reaction to the government's plans to change the status of over-the-counter herbal preparations. In the summer of 1994 the Department of Health announced that some aspects of the Medicines Act 1968 would be changed to harmonize with European Union law. At the time assurances were given that herbal medicines were unlikely to be affected, but by the autumn it was obvious that this was not the case.

Under the 1968 Act herbal medicines were exempted from the requirement of clinical testing that all orthodox pharmaceuticals had to be submitted to. This exemption would have been lost under the new regulations, with all herbal preparations subject to the requirement that they be put through clinical trials or validated through existing information. Only after this would they have received production licences. As in the 1960s, clinical trials would be impossibly expensive for the few herbal manufacturing companies to carry out. The result would therefore have been the withdrawal from sale of about 80 per cent of over-the-counter herbal preparations. Also practitioners, though not directly affected, would have been unable to obtain any materials but the crude herbs: the tinctures that have always formed the basic professional supplies would have been withdrawn along with everything else.

The NIMH and the BHMA started the campaign to save the threatened preparations in October 1994. There were two months to persuade the government to change its plans: the new legislation was to take effect from 1 January 1995. All possible sympathetic organizations were contacted with the request to make the government aware of the amount of support that herbal medicine had. Petitions were organized and submitted to the Department of Health in a matter of weeks. More letters were received there on the subject than on any other issue that can be remembered, and media coverage was generally favourable. Intense negotiations were held when it was realized how unpopular the changes would be, and in December it was announced that the plans had been changed. The government had decided that the 'traditional' techniques of preparing herbal remedies fell outside the scope of the new legislation. The campaign had been a success.

Thus we have cause for optimism about the future. Public support for herbal medicine has been amply demonstrated during the campaigns of the 1960s and the 1990s. This will be a significant factor in future negotiations with the government. Training standards have never been higher, and the number of students applying for training never greater. Research projects have been taking place that give solid evidence of the benefits of herbal remedies. Academic interest is growing too, so more research will be taking place in the future. Although there are still many challenges in the years ahead, and they may be as tough as any so far experienced, it seems at present that the position herbal medicine occupies will go from strength to strength.

HERBAL REMEDIES AND A HEALTHY LIFE

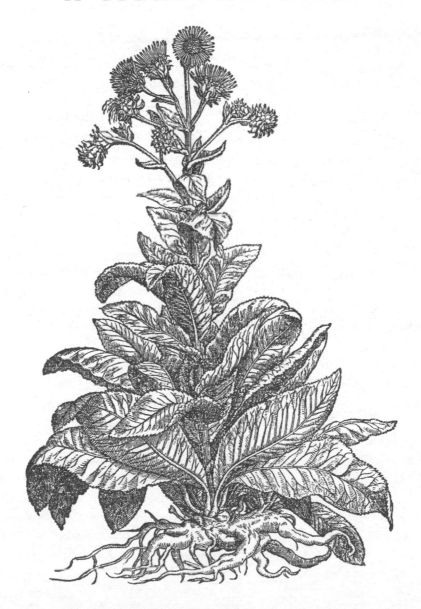

People who are interested in using herbal remedies are usually also interested in other aspects of healthy living. This chapter touches on two subjects that I think are indispensable to good health and that, if overlooked, can really lead to a general problem of feeling tired and below par much of the time. These subjects, exercise and diet, have been written about in many other books, so I will just outline my own approach in the hope that it will encourage some people to get going.

Most people leading busy lives nowadays are familiar with feelings of stress – too much traffic on the roads, pollution in the air, worries about work and money ... the list goes on and on. These are the types of stress that we are aware of being affected by, and we know the feelings of tension and short-temperedness which they provoke. There are also other types of stress on the body, which we are not so aware of, but which still take their toll. In biological terms, a stress is any change in a person's environment or situation that requires that person to change or adapt in some way as a response.

Human beings are remarkably successful at adapting to all sorts of changes, but the effort of adaptation can be costly. I think of junk-food diets and lack of exercise as stresses in this sense - they are both relatively recent changes in our way of life and we are not naturally well able to cope with them. Our bodies can survive on diets that vary from our basic requirements to some extent, and we can live without using our bodies as much as previous generations have had to, but the price is high in the long run.

It seems that to keep all our physical functions in a healthy state we need about three exercise sessions a week. This condenses the amount of steady movement that our ancestors used to get all through the day into shorter, more intense sessions. For maximum effectiveness each session should last about half an hour. If during this time you can keep moving at a steady brisk pace, but not so fast as to become completely out of breath, you will be achieving the goal of maintaining fitness and building stamina. When starting a programme of exercise, if you have any concerns about your ability to take it on, check with your medical practitioner to make sure that you can do it.

Start the exercise with some warming up and stretching exercises, and then begin the real exercise at a low pace, building up when you feel ready to take on more. If you join an exercise class these points will probably all be covered by the instructor. In the early days of an exercise programme it is quite usual to feel discouraged during it and stiff afterwards! If you can persevere you will get through this stage and start seeing some improvements in your abilities very quickly, at which point it seems much more worthwhile.

More and more evidence is suggesting that there is nothing we can take that gives us the same benefit as exercise. There is also nothing to replace its help in counteracting the harmful effects of stress. When we are active, we use up the hormones generated by stress in the way that nature intended – the 'fight or flight' nervous reactions get us ready for activity and we calm down much better after we have done some physical exercise. Anxiety and other unpleasant symptoms are definitely reduced after a good walk or swim.

Now for diet. It makes sense that if we eat the right amount of the most nutritious foods we will feel and look good. We are adapted by nature to eat a very wide range of foods, unlike many other animals, so there is plenty of scope for enjoyment! Of course different individuals might have problems eating certain foods, but these apart, the wider the range, particularly of fruit and vegetables, the better.

There are all sorts of benefits in these humble foods apart from the vitamins, minerals and fibre that we know them to contain. For instance, onions and garlic have been found to help raise the level of 'good' cholesterol – known as high density lipoprotein – in the blood; one carrot a day seems to help reduce the risk of lung cancer for a large number of people; and cranberry juice is remarkably effective at preventing urinary tract infections. Cabbage family vegetables contain a range of substances that significantly reduce the risk of developing cancers of the stomach and colon. Many other humble greens, roots, pulses, grains and salad vegetables have equally surprising benefits – we should treasure them for keeping us healthy!

Animal-based foods are not necessarily bad for the health, but because they are so much richer in fats and proteins a little goes a long way. Small amounts will help to ensure that all the required nutrients are present. Some fish extracts, notably those oils found in the flesh of brown or oily fish like mackerel, herring, trout and salmon, have a twofold benefit in that they help reduce harmful cholesterol in the bloodstream and also have an anti-inflammatory effect which helps people with arthritis and rheumatism.

If most of your diet is composed of a wide range of fairly plain-cooked wholefood ingredients, occasional treats of richer foods, sweets or snack foods won't cause any problems. It is only when such snacks replace real foods that people's health starts to suffer. I speak from experience here, having had patients who have improved as much through changes in diet as through medication, and who have stayed healthy in the long term by eating the right foods.

The Constituents and Actions of Herbs

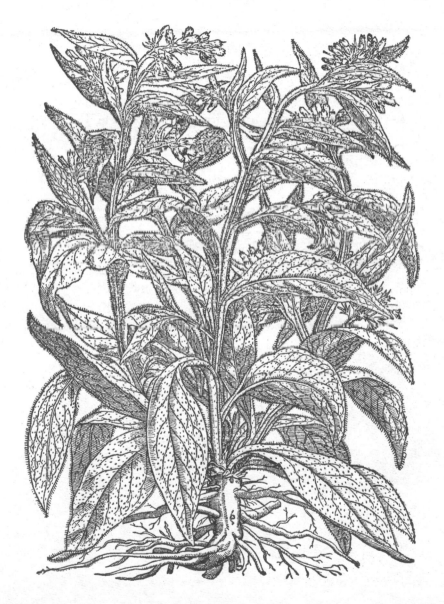

W e know something of the types of constituents found in plants that give them their main actions (although there will be thousands that might ultimately contribute to this) and the following list gives a brief outline of the most important of these.

THE CONSTITUENTS OF HERBAL REMEDIES

ALKALOIDS

These are substances containing nitrogen – the original definition meant 'vegetable alkali'. They tend to have fairly strong actions and can influence a wide range of body tissues. For instance, the caffeine found in tea and coffee is an alkaloid that stimulates the nervous system, while the 'hot' substance in chilli peppers is an alkaloid that stimulates the digestion and circulation.

BITTERS

As the name suggests, these have a characteristic taste. Don't confuse this with either sour or salty tastes, as neither of those have the same action. When any bitter taste is experienced in the mouth a message is sent via a connecting nerve to the stomach and liver, which are both stimulated to increased activity. This reflex action is the reason why certain bitter-tasting drinks are still taken, particularly in Europe, as an aperitif before meals. The drink Campari is a good example.

FLAVONOIDS

This term refers to commonly occurring vitamin-like substances that are necessary for a wide range of functions in the body. They are present in many fruits and vegetables; lemons are a good source. They are frequently found in those remedies prescribed to help problems of the circulation.

· MUCILAGES

These have a rather slippery texture that gives them their therapeutic action. They are made of starch-related substances, and when in contact with the skin or lining of the digestive system, they mimic the action of naturally produced protective mucus. This helps to calm all sorts of underlying inflammation and makes mucilages useful additions to poultices and internal preparations.

RESINS

Resins are the product of the sap of some trees. When their bark is cut the sap that seeps out hardens to form a substance that is then harvested. Most resins are used for their strong anti-infective properties. One important ingredient of the traditional remedy Friars' Balsam is very resinous, and this is responsible for the sticky deposit left in the bowl when the diluted liquid is thrown away after use – resins do not dissolve in water!

SAPONINS

These have a soapy feel to them, and take their name from the Latin word *sapo*, meaning soap. In fact the herb soapwort produces a froth when added to water; it has been used as a detergent for delicate fabrics. Other saponin-containing herbs have an influence on the stomach that produces a reflex effect in the lungs, stimulating mucus production. This can be useful if there is a problem such as a 'dry' cough where a more liquid mucus, easier to cough up, is desirable.

A different group of saponins is similar in structure to steroid-type substances. These are well known in orthodox medicine and are prescribed for many different problems. Some are controversial, as in the long term they may cause pronounced side-effects. Those that occur naturally in plants tend to have a lesser impact on the body, possibly because in the plant the saponin is one constituent among many and is present in much smaller quantities than is found in the prescribed dose of orthodox steroids. These saponins form part of many of the remedies prescribed for problems of the reproductive system, certain individual remedies having reputations as either male or female 'tonics'. Many are also useful where anti-inflammatory actions are needed.

SUGARS

These are familiar to everyone, and are derived commercially from the sap of the sugar cane or root of the sugar beet. There are small amounts of sugars in almost all leaves, as they are manufactured in this part of the plant (though this is not always obvious from the taste!). Sugars are also stored in the roots of several herbs, such as *liquorice - whose botanical name is *Glycyrrhiza*, which means 'sugar root'. This is why liquorice is traditionally used in confectionery as a natural sweetening agent. I use it in some mixtures to improve the flavour.

CAUTION

Do not take liquorice in pregnancy.
Lily of the valley should not be taken unless on the advice of
a herbal practitioner.

Some sugar-related plant constituents have wide-ranging and very useful actions. They are called glycosides. A glycoside has a sugar part joined to a different part that is usually responsible for its therapeutic action. The non-sugar parts vary enormously in structure and action.

One example is *lily of the valley. This plant has several glycosides that help to strengthen the action of the heart muscle. It is actually the non-sugar parts that do this job, but the sugar parts help their initial absorption into the body and their effectiveness in the heart muscle. Incidentally, this plant is also a very good example of the fact that whole herbs can work better than their isolated constituents. There are about six or so related glycosides in lily of the valley. When given in isolation none of them achieve the same beneficial effect as when the whole herb is given.

TANNINS

Tannins are a group of substances found widely in plants. The most familiar is ordinary tea. People who like to drink it strong will know the feeling of an astringent coating in the mouth - caused by tannin. What happens chemically is that tannins interact with proteins (of which there are thousands, in our bodies and in our foods) to harden them a process used for hundreds of years in the tanning of leather. While drinking strong tea won't have quite such a drastic action on your insides, it does produce a lesser degree of the same process. This can be very useful if the lining of the digestive system is inflamed, as one benefit of tannin-containing remedies is that they help counteract inflammation. The oversensitivity of the mucus membrane lining the digestive system can result in overactivity in the bowel, and tannins can reduce the severity of this reaction.

Externally, tannin-containing remedies can help to staunch blood loss, and reduce swellings and bruises caused by minor injuries. The old advice about putting cold teabags on overtired eyes is based on the fact that the tannin content will help to soothe the eyes. There are remedies other than tea that do a better job for most other problems, though.

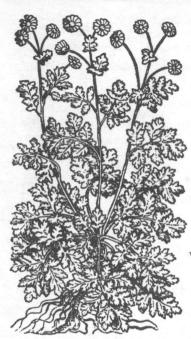

VITAMINS AND MINERALS

These are present in most plant material to some extent. Some herbs are recommended for their high nutritional content, such as nettles for iron and rosehips for Vitamin C.

VOLATILE OILS

These are plant oils that are lost very easily if the plant material is heated too much. They are the constituents that are mainly responsible for the familiar scents of our favourite garden herbs: *thyme, lavender, *sage, *rosemary and the mints are all rich in volatile oils. If you want to scent a room with one of these, place a small bunch on or near a hottish surface. The oils will evaporate quickly and the scent will fill the room. When using the plants as remedies the oils need to be conserved within the leaves (or flowers or seeds – for each individual plant the part that contains the greatest amount of oil may vary) and you should be able to detect a good scent from the material you are using. If you are making a tea from one of these plants you will get the best results by covering the tea while it is standing, otherwise some of the oils will be lost into the air with the steam.

Oils can have a large number of differing constituent molecules, in different proportions, resulting in an enormous variety of scents. They have a range of actions on the body. Most help to calm the digestion, some calm the nervous system and some are useful to help fight off infections.

CAUTION

Thyme, sage and rosemary should not be taken during pregnancy.

The Actions of Herbal Remedies

There are some traditional terms that categorize and describe the actions of herbal remedies that are little used in orthodox medicine today. The following is a list of such terms.

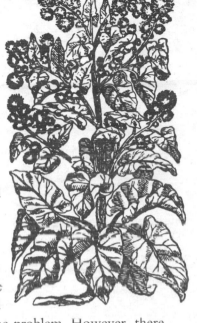

Alterative

A term applied to a large number of remedies to indicate that whichever part of the body or physical system they are used to help, they will help restore the normal function.

Anodyne

Helps relieve pain. In herbal medicine there aren't many remedies prescribed simply to ease pain, as the practitioner is more concerned with looking for and treating the causes of the problem. However, there are one or two quite harmless herbs that have a reputation for pain relief, with no associated side-effects, such as St John's wort.

Anthelmintic

This means a remedy that expels worms from the body - a very important function before the days of our current standards of hygiene. Most of the remedies with this action also have potent, possibly irritant laxative properties, so are best taken under the direction of a professional.

Antispasmodic

Muscular spasms, or cramping-type contractions, occur in connection with a range of illnesses. The painful contractions of the muscles in the intestines, known as colic, are one example. Antispasmodic remedies help to relax these muscular contractions. There are also some remedies that help to relax the muscles, such as in the calves or toes, which cause some people to wake up at night from the pain caused by cramp in them.

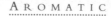

AROMATIC

This is another term for a scented remedy. It is used mainly for those remedies that are called spices, which are also used frequently as ingredients in cooking because of the flavour they impart. Generally, they are very good remedies for aiding the function of the digestive system.

ASTRINGENT

The word that describes the action of tannins. The overall result is that the affected tissues are helped to return to normal from a state of inflammation. Because these changes include a reduction in the swelling, remedies with this action are considered to have a 'contracting' influence. There are some substances other than tannins that have the same effect - think of the way neat lemon-juice makes the inside of your mouth feel!

CARMINATIVE

A remedy that calms flatulence and reduces colicky pains. Many popular herb teas and culinary spices have this action, generally due to the volatile oils they contain.

CHOLAGOGUE

A remedy that promotes the flow of bile from the liver, through the gallbladder and into the digestive tract. A healthy flow of bile is important for two reasons. First, it plays a vital role in the digestion of fats. In the Western world our consumption of fats has been rising over the last fifty years and we need efficient livers to cope (though cutting back on unnecessary fats is just as important). Second, bile contains some substances that the body is getting rid of, so it is an important channel of elimination. Cholagogues therefore have a role to play in a wide range of problems not apparently directly related to the liver. For instance, skin problems and headaches can in some cases improve greatly following the use of these remedies.

DEMULCENT

Having a soothing effect on the lining of the digestive tract or the skin. Most remedies that have this action contain mucilages. These form a protective, soothing layer over the surface of the inflamed mucus membranes or skin, allowing the normal processes of healing to proceed underneath.

DIAPHORETIC

Promoting perspiration. This is a natural skin function, though considered rather socially embarrassing nowadays. It has two valuable purposes. First, it helps to cool the body if the temperature is getting too high. Diaphoretic remedies are therefore very useful in the treatment of feverish conditions, such as minor infections like head-colds or 'flu. It should be remembered that the body produces a fever in the first place as a defence against an infection, but high fevers can be dangerous and need treating. The second function of perspiration is that it helps eliminate certain waste products through the skin. The richer supply of blood to the skin produced by diaphoretics can also make them useful in the treatment of skin problems.

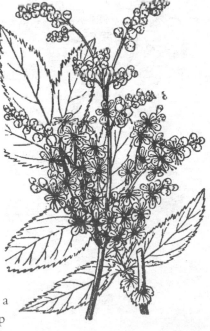

EXPECTORANT

A remedy that helps the lungs to produce a loose type of phlegm that can be coughed up easily. In cases of infection or some allergies, the membranes lining the air-passages and lungs will produce mucus as a protective strategy. When this is coughed up it takes some of the infective organisms or dust, pollen, etc. with it, thus helping to reduce the problem. Natural practitioners see that this function is very valuable and so do not try to suppress it. But problems may occur if the mucus becomes too thick to be coughed up easily, which can result in a 'dry', unproductive cough. The function of expectorants is to correct this. Their mode of action is rather interesting. Most seem to work through the effect they have on the lining of the stomach: when this is stimulated by the constituents of a herb there seems to be a reflex stimulating effect on the membranes of the lungs too, resulting in an increased production of mucus. This is a good example of how herbal medicines use those reflex pathways that already exist in the body to good effect.

Some well-known traditional expectorants are so stimulating to the stomach that in large enough doses they are actually liable to produce vomiting. At this point the stimulating effect has become so strong that it is causing irritation. Not all the expectorants have this potential for irritation, however: there are numerous examples of remedies that have a beneficial effect on the lungs but do not cause problems for the stomach.

HAEMOSTATIC

Helps staunch the flow of blood. This is relevant in minor injuries only nowadays, but was much more important in the past. Most of the remedies in this category contain tannins.

LAXATIVE

Here is one term still in common usage. Herbal laxatives are still among those most frequently prescribed by doctors. There are two broad categories. The first and most famous of all is still *senna. This is an example of a laxative that works by

stimulating an increased degree of activity in the
muscles of the bowel, as a result of the irritating
effect it has on the lining of the upper intestine.
Second, there are some remedies that work
mainly by softening and lubricating the stools,
making them pass through the digestive tract much
more easily. These remedies, such as psyllium
seeds, are far gentler than the senna-type and
are suitable for people who cannot cope with
anything in their diet that might have an
irritating effect. Generally they contain insoluble or
semi-soluble types of cellulose, which when mixed
with water form a soft gel that acts as a softening
and bulking agent. Some people find that these
remedies are more useful than an increase in the
amount of bran-fibre in their diet, as too much
bran can have an irritating effect.

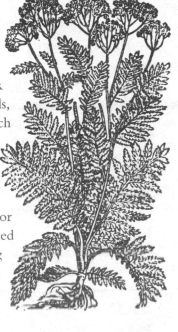

CAUTION

*Senna is best avoided during pregnancy and should only be taken under
medical supervision.*

NERVINE

This term covers a wide range of remedies that have an action on the
nervous system. Some have a stimulating effect (these I use least, as most
people's nerves are overstimulated enough by the pressures of life). Many
have a relaxing effect to various degrees. The most useful belong to a group
that can be taken by people with problems ranging from depression to
anxiety and also including physical problems such as attacks of shingles.
This group contains the remedies whose main action is to strengthen and
nourish the nerves, making them relevant to just about any problem with
the nervous system.

RUBEFACIENT

A remedy which, when applied to the skin, produces an increase in its red colouration. This is due to an increase in the local blood flow, and is usually accompanied by a sensation of increased warmth. These remedies are generally beneficial to problems such as types of rheumatism and arthritis that are worse in cold weather. The increased blood supply helps to provide more nutrients and oxygen to the affected area, while the warmth helps to activate the natural healing processes and relax tense muscles. Most of the remedies in this group are those that will cause a sensation of heat and tingling in the mouth, such as horseradish, mustard and chillies. They are used traditionally as poultices to maximize the heat imparted to the area of the body to which they are applied.

CAUTION

Rubefacient remedies should not be used on broken skin as they will cause severe pain. Also, be careful to avoid them coming into contact with the eyes or any mucus membranes.

TONIC

A somewhat general term applied to remedies that help nourish, stimulate and strengthen the functioning of a particular part of the body. There are tonics for most of the different physical systems, such as digestive, circulatory and immune system tonics.

CHAPTER 5

How to Prepare
Herbal Remedies

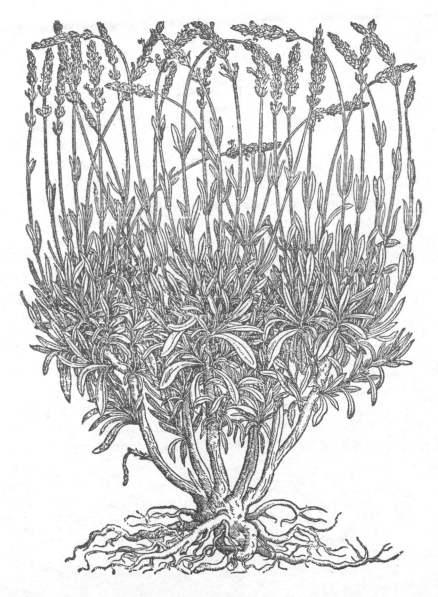

I f you visit a herb/health shop you will find various types of preparations on display. Tablets are a popular way of taking herbal remedies. They will have all the ingredients listed on the label, along with the recommended dosage. Liquids are popular for some remedies, particularly cough formulations and general tonics. Of the dried herbs available, some will be sold as teabags and others sold loose, by the 25g/1oz bag. The tablet and liquid preparations are convenient for people who don't have access to the means of preparing the dried herbs, for instance those at work or travelling. Such preparations have the added advantage that you can't taste the herb - very important for some remedies!

When you read about the different herbs in Chapter 6 you will see that for each plant the part of it which should be used is specified. For most this means the leaves and stem, but for some it is the root, bark, flowers or berries. The part used is that which has been found to have the most effective action (and therefore can be said to contain the highest amount of the plant's active constituents). There must have been a long process of observation in the past, before the techniques of scientific analysis were developed, to arrive at this knowledge. I think the research work of past herbalists who developed this body of knowledge deserves great tribute.

There is a 'timetable' of harvesting herbs, depending on which part of the plant is to be collected for use. Leaves are generally gathered in spring or summer, shortly before the plant flowers. At this time there is likely to be the highest concentration of constituents in the leaves, which are the food-manufacturing organs of the plant. If the flowers are required, these are picked before they are completely open.

Picking them any later would result in a loss of some of the constituents, which can be extremely transitory because during the period of flowering chemical changes and developments occur very rapidly. Roots of perennial plants are usually gathered in the autumn, after the top parts of the plant have died off and the important constituents have been transported down to the roots for storage over the winter. Berries are collected at an early mature stage, before they start to go soft. Seeds are harvested when they are mature, but before the dispersal mechanisms of the plant have had time to act. Some herbal remedies are in the form that would normally be recognized as seeds, but are botanically classified as fruits. The term 'fruit' is applied to any organ that contains the seeds of a plant, and does not necessarily bear any resemblance to what we think of as the fruit that we eat. This explains how the word is used in entries in Chapter 6.

Traditionally the collected material is dried in a warm but not hot environment where there is a good circulation of air, to draw off water but to conserve the other constituents. If the drying conditions are too hot, some precious volatile oils may be lost along with the water.

Buying dried herbs from a shop can pose a problem if you can't find out how long they have been there. Plant material will deteriorate if it has been stored for a long time, or if it was poorly dried in the first place. The appearance will give you some idea of the quality – avoid buying leafy material if it is faded and powdery (this rule doesn't apply to roots or barks, as even a good-quality sample can look grey and powdery!). If the scent of the plant in question is familiar to you, smell the sample to try and detect it: a good sample should still have a noticeable scent.

There is another aspect of buying herbal remedies that is rarely mentioned in other books I have come across, and that is their price. Many people assume they will not be expensive, and for most herbs this is the case. Those plants which are easy to cultivate and in plentiful supply will have a low price that reflects this. However, there are a few that have either been in such high demand in the past that they have been overcollected and are consequently becoming very rare (like echinacea and golden seal), or that have very specific cultivation requirements and so are difficult to grow (the failed attempt to grow evening primrose in Britain is an example – the climate is too cold to produce an economic yield of oil from the seeds).

So the price of these remedies is much higher than that of most others. The price of some essential oils also seems shockingly high – again reflecting the availability of raw materials and the difficulties of production. If you want to try these particular remedies, be prepared for the higher price and be very careful about buying a sample that is offered cheaply – good-quality material is unlikely to be available at less than the going rate.

When making a remedy from a dried herb the traditional quantities used are 25g (1oz) of dried herb to 570ml (1 pint) of water. This gives a rather strong-tasting preparation and I have found from experience that it often works out better to have a smaller but more palatable dose of the herb if that enables a person to enjoy taking it regularly. It is no help to have one cup of something that you can't face a second time. Try about a teaspoonful of the herb to about a cupful of water at first, and vary the strength according to your own taste. To get the medicinal benefits of the herb, the recommendation is that you take a cupful of the drink three times a day.

The simplest and most popular technique of preparation is to make a tea, also known as an infusion or tisane. This is by far the easiest means of preparing remedies for home use when using leaves or flowers; it is basically the same as making ordinary tea. In fact, the word 'tea' applies to the preparation rather than the leaves: we should ask people if they want a cup of *Camellia sinensis* when we offer them ordinary tea!

For a herb already in a teabag, simply pour water as near as possible to boiling over the bag in a cup, then cover and leave to stand for a few minutes. In this time the water will start to be coloured by the herb. It will probably not become as darkly coloured as ordinary tea, which is often selected more for colour than for flavour. Don't worry – let it stand until it has the strength of flavour you want. Most of the herbs available in teabags have a pleasant taste. They will be quite different from the taste of ordinary tea and may take a while to get used to, but I am sure that there is something for everyone among the range available in most herb/health shops. They can be flavoured with honey or fruit juices if preferred. There are many combinations of herbs now available in teabags, some for therapeutic purposes and some just for the pleasure of the taste.

With loose herbs, start by trying about a teaspoonful of the herb in a teapot and add about a cupful of boiling water to it. Leave to stand, strain, then add honey etc. if required.

If you are using plant material such as roots or stems, this is much tougher than leaves and needs longer to prepare to get the best results. The traditional technique is called a decoction. The amount of water should be about half as much again as with the teas, and the herb should be placed with the water in a pan and brought up to simmering heat on a cooker. Leave like this until the amount of water has reduced to two thirds of the original – about twenty minutes. The water should have had long enough to absorb the constituents of the plant by this time. Strain, check the taste, dilute with more water if required, then add honey or fruit juices to alter the taste if you want.

Teas and decoctions are normally to be taken three times a day to get the therapeutic benefits. The standard time to take them is after meals – which has the added advantage of being an easily remembered time when a routine can be established. The exception to this timing is those remedies that are being taken to stimulate the appetite and digestion – which obviously have to be taken before meals. About fifteen or twenty minutes before eating is an ideal time for these. Also, if the remedy is to help counteract insomnia, it will best be taken once in the evening and again about an hour before going to bed. Herbal remedies are highly suitable to being adapted to the needs of the individual, so find times to take them that suit you best. I would stress, though, that they do seem to be most successful when taken three times a day. I have found from experience that a larger dose taken twice a day generally does not give the same benefit.

Teas and decoctions account for the preparation techniques of most of the remedies that are taken internally. Each cupful should be made shortly before it is taken, as it contains no preservative. Some remedies can be preserved by being made into syrups, vinegars, etc., but that is beyond the intended scope of this book. A few plants call for some personal ingenuity in how they are best taken. For instance, with fresh garlic often the easiest thing to do is to crush the clove, mix it with honey and just swallow it as quickly as you can!

There are also several ways of preparing remedies for external application. The simplest and most useful for home use is simply to use an infusion or decoction as a lotion on the surface of the skin. This will dry without leaving any trace. Or, to expose the skin on the hands and feet to the remedy for a longer time, make a bowlful of the infusion or decoction to the same strength as for the tea. Soak the hands or feet in this when the preparation has cooled to a pleasant-feeling temperature for about ten minutes. In some parts of Europe this technique is favoured over taking the remedies by mouth. The skin is certainly a very absorbent surface: some of what you apply will be taken into the bloodstream and transported to other parts of the body. If you want to test this yourself, try rubbing garlic onto your wrists or the soles of your feet. After twenty minutes or so the smell will be coming through on your breath!

Another simply made preparation is infused oil. This is made by taking a small jar and packing into it as much of the herb as you can (getting quantities exactly proportional is less important for this product). Then pour over the herb enough oil – almond oil, for example, is easily obtained at most chemist shops – to fill the jar. Cap tightly, and keep the jar in a warm place away from bright light for a month or so. The oil will then have absorbed the properties of the herb, and will have become somewhat darker-coloured. It can now be used as an external application, gently stroked or massaged onto the skin. Four very popular herbs to prepare and use in this way are comfrey, English marigold, St John's wort and lavender. If you have access to the fresh rather than dried herbs, try using these as you are likely to get a better result: none of the constituents of the plants will have been lost. The four mentioned above are all very easy to grow, and all will make attractive additions to your garden. All except the English marigold are perennial, so once planted will give years of usefulness and pleasure. The marigold is one of the easiest annuals to grow and flowers throughout the summer: you will only need a small proportion of the flowers it produces to make the oil, and the rest will add to the colour in the garden. Make sure you have the right type of marigold – the popular African and French marigolds are completely different plants, with none of the properties of the English type.

An ointment will give a firmer consistency than an oil. There are hundreds of different ways in which it can be made, varying widely in the ingredients and techniques used. A simple and effective one is made as follows. You will need 25g (1oz) of beeswax, 150ml (1/4 pint) of sunflower oil, 25g (1oz) of the chosen herb and a small amount of tincture of benzoin. For the beeswax, the yellow variety is the best. This can be obtained from most chemist shops, or straight from a beekeeper if you know one. Ordinary cooking-grade sunflower oil is used. Soak the herb in the oil; if you are patient enough to leave this for several months you will get the best results. Otherwise the process can be speeded up by whisking the mixture in a blender for a few minutes. Either way, strain off the resulting oil and make the final amount up to 150ml by adding more sunflower oil if necessary. Melt the beeswax and stir it into the oil, adding six drops of tincture of benzoin. This is to act as a preservative; it is necessary as you will probably be keeping the ointment for a while before it is all used up. Pour the ointment into a sterile jar (you can buy either baby-bottle or beer-making equipment sterilizing liquid for this) and cap immediately. The ointment will solidify as it cools, but will still be soft enough to scoop out. Keep it in a cool place, as it will melt again if it is heated. Comfrey, chickweed, chamomile and English marigold make useful ointments.

A technique that used to be popular in the past but is less used now, though I still recommend it frequently, is *steam inhalation.

This helps reduce the discomfort and severity of a wide range of respiratory problems, from sinusitis, head–colds and laryngitis to coughs and chest infections. The basic technique is to use a very hot infusion, or to add the herbal preparation to about 570ml (1 pint) of water that is a little below boiling temperature. Constituents of the remedy will then evaporate from the liquid into the steam, which you enclose under a towel. Wait a minute or two until the most intense heat has passed, then put your head under the towel and breathe in the steam through both the nose and the mouth. The remedy is taken in with the steam and carried directly to the nasal passages and lungs, where it can start to help immediately. Also, the warm steam by itself is usually soothing to inflamed membranes. Both infectious and allergic problems can be helped in this way. Try a teaspoonful of Friar's Balsam to 570ml (1 pint) of boiling water if you have an infection (use an old bowl for this, as the insoluble constituents in the Friar's Balsam always leave a sticky deposit when you pour the water away). Use a strong tea of chamomile flowers if you have an allergic problem like hay fever.

CAUTION

Some people with asthma may find that steam is irritating to their chests. Steam inhalations should not be used in these cases.

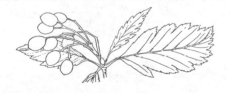

CHAPTER 6

An Alphabetical Guide
to the Remedies

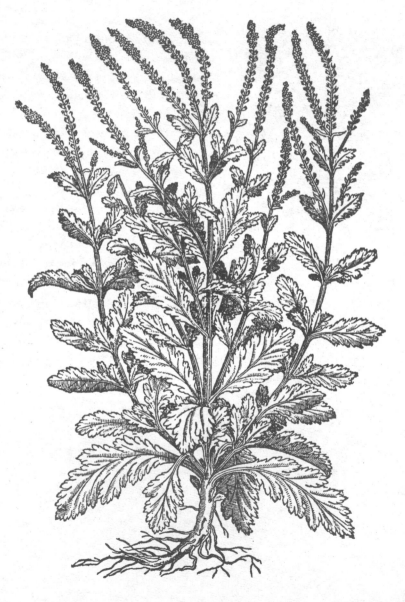

This chapter can be used in conjunction with the next (on common ailments) to find out details of how the plants recommended are helpful, or just by itself if you are interested in learning more about the fascinating properties and uses of individual herbal remedies. The format has been designed so that the key information needed to locate and identify the characteristics of the remedy are presented in a standard and easy to use way. I have not included a description of the plants, as other specialist books will do that and for those people who are considering collecting their own plants from the wild I think it is most important that a good, specialist identification guide is used. There have been tragic mistakes made occasionally, such as confusing the foxglove plant with comfrey. There is also the issue of conservation to consider. If you would like to gather fresh plants, either grow these yourself, or take from the wild only those that you know to be very common. There is no problem if you keep to those that are classed as garden weeds, such as dandelions and nettles.

C A U T I O N

Many wild plants are now legally protected. Make sure you are familiar with the law before taking anything from the wild.

You will see that as well as details about the present uses of the remedies, the entries also include historical information and even, in some cases, stories from folklore and legend. I have included this to give an idea of how important these herbs were to our ancestors, with special reference to the best known of herbalists, Nicholas Culpeper. His herbal was a great source of medical information for hundreds if not thousands of families in the past, who would have had little access to any other kind of treatment. However, it is included here for historical interest only.

CAUTION

When you are reading the entries with the intention of trying the remedies, look up all of those mentioned in the combinations, to make sure that each one is likely to suit you and the problem you are trying to deal with. Bear in mind that this information is not intended to replace the need for professional medical attention, and never try to treat an illness yourself with herbal remedies unless you are quite sure that it does not require professional diagnosis and treatment.

AGNUS-CASTUS *Vitex agnus-castus*

Family: verbenaceae. **Part used:** berries. **Constituents:** bitters, alkaloids, volatile oil. **Action:** helps regulate the pituitary gland. **Helps to:** reduce premenstrual tension, stabilize the length of the menstrual cycle, reduce menopausal problems.

Historical notes: The other common name for this plant is 'chaste tree'; it used to be thought that its berries helped to make a vow of chastity easier to maintain. It was used by the women of ancient Greece in their rituals to the goddess Ceres.

Present uses: This remedy is excellent as a regulator of female hormones, through its action on the pituitary gland (which releases hormones that control the functions of the ovaries and uterus). It seems to have a particular benefit during the last phase of the monthly cycle, which makes it particularly useful for premenstrual problems. The great majority of my women patients who have tried it for this purpose have found it helpful. It can alleviate both the physical problems, like fluid retention and fatigue, and the emotional ones. Take the berries as a tea, using about a quarter of a teaspoonful at each dose. Most women find they only need to take it once a day, in the morning, but it can be taken up to three times daily if this proves necessary to get the benefit.

AGRIMONY *Agrimonia eupatoria*

Family: rosaceae. **Part used:** leaves and stem. **Constituents:** volatile oil, bitters, tannins. **Action:** gentle astringent to digestive system, bitter tonic. **Helps to:** reduce discomfort and overactivity of bowel-function in 'upsets' of digestive system.

Historical notes: The herb is named after the Greek word used for herbs that were healing to the eyes *(argemone),* and after King Mithridates Eupator, who was famous for his interest in herbal remedies. Used since Anglo-Saxon times in Britain, it had a reputation for treating wounds, snake-bites, haemorrhages, coughs and diarrhoea.

Present uses: Prepare this as a tea. It is an excellent remedy for problems of the digestive system where there is irritation and overactivity of the bowels. Where there is an infection it will help to reduce the discomfort of the body's reaction to this without actually inhibiting it. (Bear in mind that the functions of vomiting and diarrhoea are to protect you against anything harmful you may have swallowed. They help to get it out of the body as quickly as possible. It is only when these reactions are very severe or prolonged that they become a problem in themselves.) Some people may have sensitivities to certain foods which cause irritation and reflex overactivity: agrimony will be useful here.

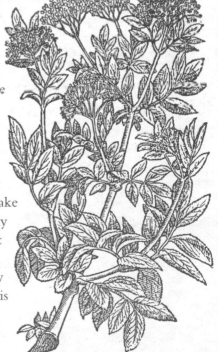

Combines well with: meadowsweet, mixed in equal parts with agrimony for maximum benefit for stomach problems. Take slippery elm powder (which is probably more palatable taken as a separate drink as it is prepared differently) for both stomach and bowel problems. Combine agrimony with any of the carminatives if flatulence is part of the problem.

Culpeper says: *'It helpeth the cholic, cleanseth*

the breast, and relieves the cough. A draught of the decoction, taken warm before the fit, first removes and then relieves the tertian or quartan ague. The leaves and seed, taken in wine, stay the bloody flux; outwardly being applied, being stamped with old swine's grease, it helpeth old sores, cancers, and inveterate ulcers. It draweth forth thorns, splinters of wood, nails, or any such thing gotten into the flesh.'

ANGELICA *Angelica archangelica*

Family: umbelliferae. **Part used:** leaf and root. The stems and seeds are used in confectionery and culinary flavouring. **Constituents:** volatile oil, bitters, astringent substance. **Action:** warming and stimulating to digestive system, lungs and circulation. Carminative, expectorant, and improves the body's ability to cope with problems made worse by cold weather.

Historical notes: The use of angelica goes back to antiquity: it has always been considered of sovereign value. It features in various pagan and old Christian stories and folk practices. The root had a reputation for helping against the bite of poisonous animals and epidemic diseases, and for 'comforting the heart blood and spirits'.

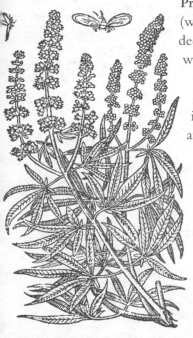

Present uses: Prepare the leaves as a tea, or the root (which is what I personally use more) as a decoction. Angelica can be used in cases where a warming and stimulating action is desirable but where the 'hot' remedies such as chillies and ginger are too irritating to the stomach. Angelica is much gentler and better tolerated. It is aromatic, particularly the root, which has a very pleasant scent; it aids the efficiency of the digestion and it reduces problems like flatulence and colic. It is a good support for other cough remedies, as the warming properties help the lungs to resist the ill effects of cold weather. Breathing in cold, damp air in winter can often irritate an already ailing chest, as many people in Britain who have chronic chest problems will know. Cold weather can irritate many other problems, such as arthritis and eczema, especially when the affected area is exposed to the cold.

Combines well with: other relevant remedies against the cold, depending on the particular nature of a person's symptoms.

Culpeper says: *'Angelica signifies the angelical or angel-like herb. The water distilled out of the roots is good against gnawing and pains of the belly occasioned by cold. Moreover it is good for diseases of the lungs and for the stranguary. It expelleth the wind that is in the body and eases the pain that cometh from the same.'*

ANISEED *Pimpinella anisum*

Family: umbelliferae. **Part used:** whole fruit. **Constituents;** volatile oil, sugar, mucilage. **Action:** aromatic, carminative, expectorant. **Helps to:** soothe the digestion, calm flatulence, relieve chest problems.

Historical notes: Aniseed has been cultivated in Mediterranean countries since the time of the Romans and has been used in Britain since the fourteenth century. It is a traditional ingredient in cakes, liqueurs and confectionery, and folklore held that it was helpful in keeping away the 'evil eye'.

Present uses: Prepare this as a tea. It makes a pleasant drink following a meal to help reduce discomfort, flatulence and colic. It is also useful as an accessory remedy for most chest problems, as it helps to loosen tight phlegm and soothe a hard, unproductive type of cough.

Combines well with: any relevant remedies to help the digestive system or the chest. Its well-known sweet taste and scent will improve the flavour of other herbs – an important aspect when giving remedies to children.

ARNICA *Arnica montana*

Family: compositae. **Part used:** flowers. **Constituents:** volatile oil, tannin, bitter substance. **Action:** promotes the dispersal of blood that has leaked into the tissues. **Helps to:** speed up the healing of bruises.

Present uses: There is only one function that arnica has, but for this it is an outstanding remedy. It can be obtained in most herb or health shops in the form of a cream or ointment, and is an excellent treatment for minor injuries where swelling and bruising are concerned. A very useful remedy to have to hand when involved in sports activities, it also makes a good application to chilblains to promote healing.

Combines well with: witch-hazel, which also helps to reduce the pain and swelling of minor injuries.

C A U T I O N

Arnica should never be taken internally or applied to broken skin - it could have dangerous consequences. Used externally on unbroken skin it is harmless.

B E A R B E R R Y *Arctostaphyllos uva-ursi*

Family: ericaceae. **Part used:** leaf. **Constituents:** flavonoids, acids, tannins, hydroquinones. **Action:** urinary antiseptic, astringent. **Helps to:** reduce urinary infections.

Historical notes: Bearberry has been used in the tanning industries of Sweden and Russia because of its high tannin content. Its medicinal use was recorded by the Myddfai physicians of Wales as far back as the thirteenth century.

Present uses: Bearberry is an excellent anti-infective remedy for problems like cystitis. This action only affects the urinary system, as the active ingredient, thought to be hydroquinone, is formed after a precursor substance enters the urinary system for excretion. It works much better if the urine is alkaline, which can be achieved by a change in the diet to reduce the intake of meat and cereals, and to increase that of fruit and vegetables.

Combines well with: soothing diuretics like *horsetail, to clear an infection and reduce discomfort.

C A U T I O N

Bearberry should not be taken during pregnancy or by people with kidney problems.
Horsetail should not be taken by people with heart problems.

BENZOIN

Styrax benzoin

Family: styraceae. **Part used:** gum (resin). **Constituents:** benzoic acid. **Action:** antiseptic, expectorant. **Helps to:** improve the condition of the lungs in coughs and chest infections.

Historical notes: It has been used for hundreds of years in perfumes and pomanders, and was burnt in the house to create a pleasant scent.

Present uses: The resin is obtained by making cuts in the bark of the styrax tree (found in Sumatra, Java and Thailand). Interestingly, the normal constituents of the sap of the tree do not contain the same substances as the resin, and it may be that the liquid that oozes out and hardens to form the antiseptic resin is specially produced by the tree to protect it against attack by harmful organisms. It is an important ingredient in Friar's Balsam, which is easily obtained at chemist shops as it is a recognized pharmaceutical product.

The technique of *steam inhalation used to be very familiar in homes, but has tended to die out now. It is well worth reviving, as it can bring great relief to the symptoms of sinusitis, throat infections and chesty coughs. The antiseptic and soothing properties of the balsam are taken in with the steam and transported directly to the membranes they benefit. This can bring a rapid feeling of relief. Phlegm is loosened and breathing becomes easier. It can also help to reduce the severity of problems like head-colds if the inhalation is performed as soon as the infection is felt to be coming on.

CAUTION

Some people with asthma may find that steam is irritating to their chests. Steam inhalations should not be used in these cases.

BLACK HAW

Viburnum prunifolium

Family: caprifoliaceae. **Part used:** root bark. **Constituents:** glycosides, tannin, resin, acids. **Action:** antispasmodic, particularly for the uterus. **Helps to:** reduce painful contractions of the uterine muscle, may help to reduce heavy periods.

Historical notes: This shrub is very closely related to the guelder rose, also known as cramp bark. Of the two, black haw has always been the more used in North America, while in Britain cramp bark is probably the more familiar.

Present uses: Black haw is one of the most widely applicable remedies for a range of menstrual problems. Pain or discomfort during menstruation is about the most widespread of all problems – most women experience it to some degree at some time. Black haw, made as a tea at the standard strength, is the best remedy for treating this. Women who suffer severe pain every cycle should start to take it three times a day, from a few days before their period is due until the time the pain is usually over. It may also help reduce heavy blood loss, and is helpful during the menopause if irregular bleeding becomes a problem.

Combines well with: *motherwort for any of the problems mentioned, and with chamomile or St John's wort as well for painful periods.

CAUTION

Do not take motherwort if you may be pregnant.

BLADDERWRACK

Fucus vesiculosus

Family: fucaceae. **Part used:** whole plant, known botanically as the thallus. **Constituents.** volatile oil, bitter substances, mucilage, minerals including sodium, potassium, iodine. **Action:** nutritional and a stimulant to the thyroid gland. A mineral supplement. **Helps to:** increase thyroid activity, restore depleted minerals.

Historical notes: It is traditionally used as a garden fertilizer by coastal communities, as it is very rich in minerals. Iodine was originally obtained by the burning of bladderwrack; this was an important industry at one time.

Present uses: This remedy is not very palatable to most people, so although it is available in powdered form I would recommend tablets as the easiest way of taking it. It is used mainly as a nutritional supplement and stimulant for the thyroid gland. This gland, located at the notch at the top of the breast-bone, produces a hormone that regulates the rate at which the body uses energy. If it becomes underactive a person will feel slow, sluggish and cold and will gain weight very easily without in fact overeating. In some parts of the world iodine is lacking in the soil and therefore also lacking in locally grown produce. Switzerland used to be such an area, and underactive thyroid problems were very common there because the gland cannot make the hormone without iodine. The condition known as 'goitre' (a prominent swelling in the notch above the breast-bone) was the result. There can be other causes of goitre as well as iodine deficiency, but a bladderwrack supplement is well worth trying in any case. Some people may have a deficiency of other minerals that can be corrected with bladderwrack: it is a valuable addition to the diet for those who don't like to add *salt to their food.

CAUTION

Bladderwrack is not recommended for people on a medical salt-free diet. It also should not be taken in pregnancy.

BONESET *Eupatorium perfoliatum*

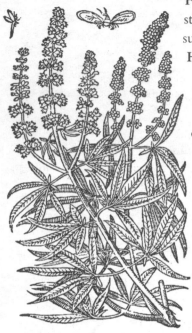

Family: compositae. **Part used:** leaves and stem. **Constituents:** volatile oil, bitter, resin, sugar. **Action:** diaphoretic, expectorant, tonic.

Helps to: reduce the severity of symptoms associated with head-colds, 'flu and catarrh.

Historical notes: It was used as the main treatment for many different diseases if they caused a fever. The name comes from the use it was put to in helping to relieve a type of 'flu in the United States during the nineteenth century, where the pain in the limbs was so bad that the disease was known as 'break-bone fever'.

Present uses: Take this as a tea: as well as being the traditional technique for leaves, taking boneset in the form of a hot drink seems to add to its benefits. It is invaluable in cases of head-colds, 'flu, chesty coughs, minor feverish illnesses and catarrh.

Combines well with: *elecampane and white horehound for coughs and chest problems; and with ground ivy for catarrh problems. Also mix it with yarrow or hyssop to help reduce a fever; and with echinacea to help fight off a respiratory infection.

CAUTION

Elecampane should not be taken in pregnancy.

BURDOCK *Arctium lappa*

Family: compositae. **Part used:** root. **Constituents:** sugars, mucilage, glycosides, resin, volatile oils. **Action:** alterative, diuretic, diaphoretic.

Helps to: improve the condition of skin infections, boils and abscesses, etc.

Historical notes: Burdock is traditionally termed a 'blood purifier' and has been used for all types of skin problems, both taken internally and used as a poultice or lotion on the affected area of skin. The seeds are credited by traditional American practitioners with having the ability to improve the texture of a dry skin by restoring its normal oil content. It was also thought to be helpful 'against the bites of serpents and mad dogs'. The traditional drink made from dandelion and burdock would have been a good tonic and helped elimination through the liver and kidneys.

Present uses: Make a decoction from the root. Burdock is used mainly for skin problems such as acne and recurrent boils, and for recurrent mouth ulcers, gingivitis, etc. I also use it to help the body recover from internal infections or other problems where waste products need to be removed by the circulation of the blood, for disposal by the kidneys and liver.

Combines well with: liver remedies such as yellow dock root. *Celery seeds will add to its ablity to expel waste products via the kidneys.

Culpeper says: *'A dram of the roots taken with pine kernels, helpeth them that spitteth foul, mattery and bloody phlegm; the leaves applied to the places troubled with the shrinking of the sinews or arteries, gives much ease. The juice of the leaves, given to drink with old wine, doth wonderfully help the bitings of serpents. The juice of the leaves taken with honey, provoketh urine and remedieth the pain of the bladder. The seed being drunk in wine forty days together, doth wonderfully help the sciatica.'*

C A U T I O N

Celery seeds should not be taken in pregnancy.

CARAWAY *Carum carvi*

Family: umbelliferae. **Part used:** seeds. **Constituents:** volatile oil, tannin. **Action:** carminative. **Helps to:** improve the digestion, reduce flatulence and colic.

Historical notes: Used since Roman times, this plant has at times been considered a vegetable as well as a herb. The young roots have been eaten and considered by some to be superior in flavour to parsnips. It may have been introduced to the West by the Arabs, as its name derives from the Arabic word *karawya*, by which it is still known in the East. It was a very popular English culinary spice by the Elizabethan age. Sweets known as 'comfits' were originally made by coating caraway seeds with layers of sugar. Adding the seeds to rye bread is a popular European custom. Caraway also formed an ingredient in love-potions as it was thought to promote fidelity, and was believed to prevent the theft of any object in which it was placed.

Present uses: Take as a tea. It possesses similar properties to aniseed in aiding the digestion, but does not have a similar reputation for helping chest problems. The taste is sweeter and less pungent than aniseed, and may be preferable to some people for this reason. It will help to reduce digestive discomfort and flatulence and to relieve colic pains. It may help to allay nausea and diarrhoea, and is often more palatable than other remedies for people with these problems.

Combines well with: chamomile to make a pleasant-tasting drink to help the digestion and ease nausea. Mix with agrimony for a more effective anti-diarrhoea treatment.

Culpeper says: *'The root is better food than the parsnip and is pleasant and comforting to the stomach, aiding digestion; the seed is a remedy for all the cold griefs* *of the head and stomach and the powder of the seed takes away black and blue spots of blows and bruises.'*

CARDAMOM

Elettaria cardamomum

Family: zingiberaceae. **Part used:** seeds. **Constituents:** volatile oil, mucilage. **Action:** carminative. **Helps to:** improve the digestion, reduce flatulence and colic.

Historical notes: Used traditionally as an ingredient in the perfume industry. Also a well-known culinary spice, used to flavour tea and coffee in the Middle East and also used as an ingredient in the Middle Eastern mixture of spices commonly chewed after meals.

Present uses: Crush the seeds and make them into a tea. This pungent, sweet-flavoured spice has similar properties to caraway. The large seeds can be made into a tea or chewed whole if you like the flavour, in which case the sense of warmth they impart will be much stronger. They will help the digestion and ease flatulence and colic.

CASCARA *Rhamnus purshiana*

Family: rhamnaceae. **Part used:** bark. **Constituents:** anthraquinones (a group of glycosides). **Action:** laxative. **Helps to:** produce an easier bowel-motion.

Present uses: Take the bark as a decoction. Alternatively, several commercial preparations containing cascara will be available from either health/herb shops or chemist shops. This must be, along with *senna, one of the best known of all herbal remedies! It has a gentler action than senna, and causes less griping discomfort. It is one of the laxatives that exerts an irritant action, however, and thus stimulates the muscles of the bowel to increased activity. There is a time lapse of eight hours before it is effective, so is recommended to be taken last thing at night. It is not suitable for people who already feel a great deal of tension in the abdomen, or who are already experiencing colic-type pains. These symptoms show that there is an existing condition of excess tightening in the muscles; increasing this still further will not be beneficial.

Combines well with: any of the carminative remedies to reduce the risk of griping pains. You may get a successful result with a smaller dose of cascara if you take psyllium seeds as well.

CAUTION

Cascara should not be taken during pregnancy.
Senna is best avoided during pregnancy and should always be taken under medical supervision.

CATMINT *Nepeta cataria*

Family: labiateae. **Part used:** leaves and flowering tops. **Constituents:** volatile oil. **Action:** carminative, diaphoretic, antispasmodic. **Helps to:** aid the digestion, reduce the symptoms of a fever; may help with headaches.

Historical notes: Folklore says that 'if the root be chewed it will make the most quiet person fierce and quarrelsome'. There is also a story about a hangman who could never bring himself to do his job without first taking a drink of catmint tea! The tea was taken as a regular drink by peasants in Britain before the habit of drinking oriental tea became popular.

Present uses: Take as a hot tea to get the best antifever action. This is one of the most useful remedies for feverish colds, particularly in children, as it has a gentle calming effect as well as working to reduce a high temperature. It will also help to settle the digestion. Mix it with boneset for feverish colds.

Combines well with: limeflowers, with which it can be mixed when making a remedy to give to children.

Culpeper says: *'Nep [catmint] is generally used by women, being taken either inwardly or outwardly, either alone or with other convenient herbs, in a decoction to bathe them, or to sit over the hot fumes thereof, and, by frequent use thereof, it taketh away barrenness, and the wind, and the pains of the mother.'*

CAYENNE
Capsicum minimum

Family: solanaceae. **Part used:** fruit.
Constituents: alkaloids, fatty acids. **Action:** stimulant to digestion and circulation, rubefacient. **Helps to:** impart warmth and vitality to a range of functions in the body.

Historical notes: Used traditionally in the East in cooking. It has a reputation for 'warding off diseases' generally. Highly prized by herbalists in the past, particularly the American practitioners of the nineteenth century who used it to increase the 'heat' within the body on the principle that the cause of much disease lay in obstructions to heat. A typical treatment would be to give patients a very hot bath, dose them with cayenne and afterwards give them a very strong laxative – these herbalists had a robust approach to their work!

Present uses: Take as a low-strength tea (the effect on the mouth is overpowering otherwise!). The highly stimulating effect this remedy has locally is well known from the way that curries containing it make the lining of the mouth tingle. It has a stimulating effect on the stomach and digestion generally. It also stimulates the circulation, helping to reduce the risk of chills in people who have been exposed to too much cold or damp weather. It will help improve the resistance of the lungs against the effects of cold, damp weather for people who have chronic lung disease, and is useful in the early stages of head-colds or other catarrhal problems.

When applied externally in the form of an oil or ointment cayenne helps stimulate blood flow through the underlying area. This is a useful aid to healing in a range of illnesses, particularly those that are adversely affected by cold weather. The tea can also be used in hand- or footbaths.

CAUTION

Cayenne can be irritating to sensitive mucus membranes and skin. Be careful not to get it in your eyes. Do not apply to broken skin, or to conditions that feel hot and inflamed to start with.

Combines well with: several other remedies, with which it is frequently used to make them more fitting for the adverse effects of winter weather e.g. with boneset for colds and 'flu. Mix it with other more palatable carminative remedies for digestive problems. It combines well with comfrey as an application for arthritis or to muscular injuries and inflammation.

Culpeper says: *'For it doth not only give good taste or relish to the meat or sauce, but is found to be very good both to discuss the wind and the cholic in the body: it is of singular service to be used with flatulent or windy diet. Being mixed with nitre and applied, it takes away the morphew, and all freckles, spots, marks, and discolourings of the skin; applied with hen's grease, it dissolves all cold imposthumes and carbuncles.'*

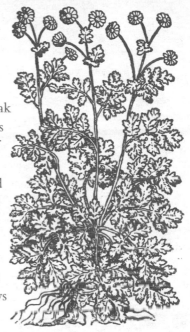

Celandine (Greater)
Chelidonium majus

Family: papaveraceae. **Part used:** fresh juice.
Constituents: alkaloids (enzymes that break down protein). **Action:** proteolytic (breaks down proteins) in the abnormal skin tissue of warts. **Helps to:** remove warts.

Historical notes: This remedy has been used extensively in the past for problems associated with the liver, though I do not recommend it to be taken internally. Its name comes from Roman times, after the Greek word *chelidon* meaning a swallow, as the flowers appeared at the same time of year that the swallows arrived. The juice was used in a dilute form for treating films over the surface of the eye, and was reported by the herbalist Gerard 'to sharpen the sight, for it cleanseth and consumeth away slimie things that cleave about the ball of the eye and hinder the sight' – a very good description of the action of the protein-destroying enzyme. The yellow colour of the juice was taken to indicate that it was a remedy for jaundice and liver problems.

Present uses: This is the most reliable remedy I have found for getting rid of warts. The fresh juice is needed for this, so you must find a growing plant for treatment. This is not difficult, as it grows widely as a weed, even in the middle of cities. If you cultivate a plant in your garden it will seed itself prolifically. The treatment itself couldn't be easier – simply snap off a piece of stem, wait a minute or so for a drop of juice to appear at the end and then dab it onto the wart. Repeat this twice a day for two weeks and the wart will go. I have tried this numerous times on family and friends and it has never caused discomfort. It is also generally well tolerated by children because of its novelty (it is much less unpleasant than the conventional techniques of removing warts). The appearance of the warts during treatment is rather unsightly as they turn a dark brownish colour, but this is the only disadvantage.

Culpeper says: *'Let it be gathered when the Sun is in Leo and the Moon is in Aries, then you may make it into an oil or ointment, which you please, to annoint sore eyes with; I can prove it from my own experience that the most desperate sore eyes hath been cured by this medicine only. The herb or root, being boiled in white wine, with a few aniseeds therein, and drunk, openeth obstructions of the liver and gall, helpeth the yellow jaundice and often using it helps the dropsy, the itch, and those who have old sores in their legs, or other parts of their body.'*

C A U T I O N

Greater celandine is not recommended to be taken internally.

C E L A N D I N E (L E S S E R)
R a n u n c u l u s f i c a r i a

Family: ranunculaceae. **Part used:** leaves. **Constituents:** astringent substances. **Action:** astringent. **Helps to:** ease haemorrhoids.

Historical notes: The old name of 'pilewort' for this plant succinctly sums up its value. It has been used since the Middle Ages for this problem, the explanation being that 'if you dig up the root of it you will perceive the perfect image of the disease commonly called the piles'. This refers to the tiny underground bulb-like structures by which the plant reproduces. They were thought to resemble the appearance of haemorrhoids and thus, according to the Doctrine of Signatures (the medieval belief that a plant's use was indicated by its appearance), were to be used to treat this problem.

Present uses: As in the past, lesser celandine is still considered the sovereign remedy for haemorrhoids. You can make a double-strength tea of the leaves and use this as a lotion, or buy a commercially available ointment ready-made. Alternatively, mix the finely powdered herb into witch-hazel gel - the astringent action of both remedies makes an excellent combination to reduce discomfort and shrink the haemorrhoids. Use the preparations at least twice a day, or more frequently if they bring a noticeable feeling of relief.

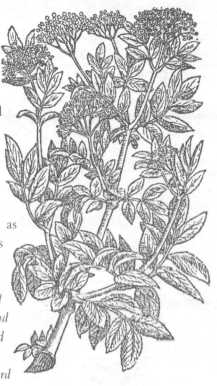

Combines well with: witch-hazel, which has already been mentioned as another effective remedy. Marigold is also used with lesser celandine for its soothing and healing actions.

Culpeper says: *'It is certain from good experience, that the decoction of the leaves and roots doth wonderfully help the piles and haemorrhoids, as also kernels by the ears and throat, called the King's evil, or any other hard wens or tumours.'*

CELERY *Apium graveolens*

Family: umbelliferae. **Part used:** seeds. **Constituents:** volatile oil, flavonoids, possible alkaloids; *stem and root*: minerals. **Action:** diuretic, carminative. **Helps to:** improve efficiency of kidney function, improve digestion.

Historical notes: The whole plant has been in use medicinally since the time of Hippocrates, the 'father of medicine' who lived in Greece more than 2,000 years ago. Its properties as a digestive stimulant and diuretic have been known since then, and its use as a vegetable is widespread throughout America, Europe and Africa.

Present uses: Make the seeds into a tea, or take the commercially produced tablets. This remedy is the best one to take at the onset of rheumatic or arthritic problems. It seems to help the kidneys in their work of removing waste products from the body. It is particularly successful at treating gout, which is due specifically to the accumulation of too much uric acid in the affected joints. Celery helps to eliminate this acid through the kidneys.

The need for improved elimination through the kidneys may underlie a wider range of problems, and celery may in this way help in cases of skin problems. It is also useful in infections of the bladder, possibly helping to reduce the infection as well as soothing the inflamed tissue and supporting kidney function. Celery stems as a food will have a similar though weaker action, as the highest concentration of active ingredients is found in the seeds. **Combines well with:** nettles to help rheumatism and gout.

C A U T I O N

Do not take celery seeds in pregnancy.

C H A M O M I L E (G E R M A N)
Chamomilla recutita
(until recently known as
Matricaria recutita)
Family: compositae. **Part used:** flowers. **Constituents:** volatile oil, mucilage, bitters, flavonoids. **Action:** carminative, antispasmodic, anti-inflammatory, nervine. **Helps to:** allay problems of the digestive system, calm nervous tension, soothe inflammation.

Historical notes: The plant's name comes from the Greek words *kamai* and *melon*, which mean 'on the ground' and 'apple', because the scent of the flowers is similar to that of apples. The Spanish word for it, *manzanilla*, means 'little apple'. Chamomile was traditionally referred to by gardeners as the plants' physician, and was thought to bring ailing plants back to health if planted near them. It is a tough herb, resisting damage when it is trodden on, and has made an excellent fragrant lawn plant. It was also used as one of the sweet strewing herbs on floors in the Middle Ages. Herbalists in the past designated it the 'mother of the gut' because of its use in combating digestive problems. Children can be encouraged to drink chamomile by telling them the Beatrix Potter story where Peter Rabbit is given it by his mother after coming home from his adventures in Mr McGregor's garden.

Present uses: There are two types of chamomile: German and Roman. The appearance of the flowers is quite different but the constituents and actions are very similar. It is almost always the German type that is available in Britain. The sweet-smelling daisy-like flowers must be the best-known of all our favourite herbs. Chamomile teabags are now becoming available even in supermarkets - a sure sign of its growing popularity.

Take the tea internally for just about any problem associated with the digestive system. It is particularly important to cover the tea when it is standing because some of the most active constituents of the oil are formed during this process, and will be lost otherwise. Chamomile is especially useful where stress is the cause of the problem, as it has a gentle relaxing action too. It suits children very well as a calming and anti-inflammatory remedy.

Externally, the tea can be used as a lotion on rashes and problems such as eczema -

some of its constituents have been found to
be as effective as steroid creams in
reducing inflammation. It is available
as a cream from most chemist shops,
marketed as a remedy for cracked or
inflamed skin.

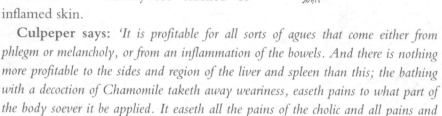

Culpeper says: *'It is profitable for all sorts of agues that come either from phlegm or melancholy, or from an inflammation of the bowels. And there is nothing more profitable to the sides and region of the liver and spleen than this; the bathing with a decoction of Chamomile taketh away weariness, easeth pains to what part of the body soever it be applied. It easeth all the pains of the cholic and all pains and torments of the belly.'*

Combines well with: any of the other carminative remedies if you dislike the taste by itself. Try the cream applied alternately with witch-hazel to soothe inflammation of the skin.

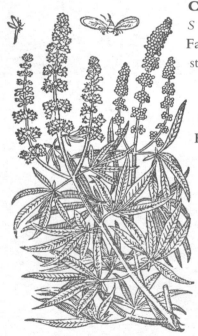

CHICKWEED
Stellaria media

Family: caryophylaceae. **Part used:** leaves and stem. **Constituents:** saponins. **Action:** anti-inflammatory, demulcent, antipruritic (reduces itching). **Helps to:** heal the skin, reduce inflammation, reduce itching of the skin.

Historical notes: This common garden weed has always been known as a favourite of chickens and caged birds, hence its name. The herbalist Gerard says 'little birds in cadges (especially Linnets) are refreshed with the lesser Chickweed when they loath their meat'. It has also been eaten raw or cooked as a vegetable, and certainly is a good source of iron. The Vitamin C content made it a useful remedy for scurvy. Externally, it was used either in a poultice made of the fresh leaves or

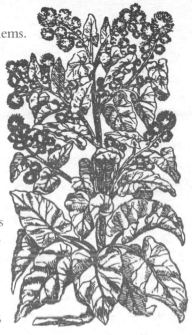

as an ointment for a wide range of problems. Stubborn skin ulcers were said to respond to such applications, and the function of internal organs was said to improve if the poultice was placed over them.

Present uses: Modern herbalists hold chickweed in just as high regard as previous generations for its soothing effect on the skin. There is nothing else as valuable to try as a tea, taken by mouth and applied as a lotion, where the skin is damaged, inflamed or itching. Saponins are known to have some anti-inflammatory properties, but the action of chickweed as a whole seems more subtle and complex as it helps to promote healing as well as calming inflammation. When used as an ointment, it has also proved useful to many of my female patients who have the type of vaginal irritation associated with low oestrogen levels. To get its benefit in a case of extensive eczema, a tea of chickweed, preferably the fresh plant, can be added to the bathwater.

Combines well with: comfrey externally to promote rapid healing of minor injuries, and with chamomile applied to patches of eczema.

Culpeper says: '*The herb bruised, or the juice applied, with cloths or sponges dipped therein is effectual for all redness in the face, wheals, itch and scabs, the juice being either simply used or boiled in hog's grease; the same helpeth cramps, convulsions and palsies and is of good effect to ease the pains and heat and sharpness of blood in the piles.*'

CLIVERS
Galium aparine

Family: rubiaceae. **Part used:** leaves and stem. **Constituents:** glycosides, tannins, acids. **Action:** diuretic, alterative, supports lymphatic function. **Helps to:** reduce fluid retention, improve efficiency of kidneys and lymphatic system (tissue cleansing and fighting infection).

Historical notes: This plant has been traditionally used as a 'blood purifier', and is an ingredient in the combination of young fresh leaves that were customarily taken as a tea in the springtime to help cleanse the body. The alternative names are goosegrass or sticky grass. The long tough strands it forms in the summer have been used to form sieves and strainers and were traditionally used for straining milk in Sweden.

Present uses: It is valuable for a wide range of problems. If the fresh plant is available, use it: the dried form seems much less effective. Make a tea of the whole herb (taking off the small leaves would be very tedious). Try this remedy to help with skin problems, where both the removal and elimination of waste products are desirable. It is also useful for infections, particularly where the lymph glands are involved (these glands react to an infection by swelling and trapping it rather than allowing it to spread further into the body).

Combines well with: stinging nettles and dandelion leaves, which were traditionally used with clivers for a 'spring cleanser'. The three were picked when young and tender, and made into a tea to help the elimination of waste products that might have accumulated over the winter when outdoor activities and exercise were reduced. These remedies are also a good source of minerals. Alternatively, combine clivers with red clover to make a tea to help clear skin problems.

Culpeper says: *'The juice of the herb, and the seed taken in wine, help those that are bitten with an adder, by preserving the heart from the venom. It is often taken in broth to keep those lean and lank that are apt to grow fat. The juice of the leaves or the leaves a little bruised, and applied to any bleeding wound, stayeth the bleeding. It is a good remedy in the Spring, eaten, being first chopped small and boiled well in water gruel, to cleanse the blood and strengthen the liver.'*

CLOVER SEE RED CLOVER

CLOVES *Eugenia caryophylla*
Family: myrtaceae. **Part used:** dried flower buds. **Constituents:** volatile oil. **Action:** aromatic, carminative, stimulant. **Helps to:** calm the digestion, reduce flatulence and colic.
Historical notes: This spice has been known in the West since about the fifth century. Its pungent aroma and flavour are very familiar from its use as a culinary herb, and the oil extracted from it used to be a well-known treatment for toothache.

Present uses: I think it is best limited to culinary use as there is some question about the safety of its constituents, if taken long term or in large doses.

COLTSFOOT
Tussilago farfara
Family: compositae. **Part used:** flowers and leaves. **Constituents:** mucilage, bitters, glycosides, minerals, notably zinc. **Action:** expectorant. **Helps to:** ease dry coughs, loosen tight phlegm.
Historical notes: One old name for coltsfoot was 'filius ante patrem', meaning 'the son before the father'. This was because, unlike most plants, coltsfoot produces its flowers before its leaves. It has always been valued for its use in chest problems and is about the best-known of

all cough remedies. It is available in several commercial herbal cough mixtures, and used to be popular as a confection known as coltsfoot rock.

Present uses: A very effective remedy as a tea for dry, unproductive coughs. It will often loosen phlegm and soothe irritation in the chest when nothing else works. It can also help reduce the severity of asthma problems. Children generally respond well to this remedy.

Combines well with: *elecampane or white horehound in a mixture for chesty coughs. Add aniseed to improve the flavour.

CAUTION

Coltsfoot has recently been found to contain a small amount of certain alkaloids thought to be dangerous if taken in large quantities. Although there have been no cases where the whole plant has been shown to be dangerous, long-term use of it is not advised.

Do not take elecampane in pregnancy.

Culpeper says: *'The fresh leaves, or juice, or a syrup made thereof, is good for a hot dry cough, for wheezings and shortness of breath: the dry leaves are best for those that have thin rheums and distillations upon their lungs, causing a cough.'*

COMFREY

Symphytum officinale

Family: boraginaceae. **Part used:** leaves and root. **Constituents:** allantion, tannin, resins. **Action:** demulcent, astringent; promotes rapid tissue-healing. **Helps to:** heal minor wounds and ulcers.

Historical notes: The alternative common names, 'knitbone' and 'consolida', indicate that this plant has a long history of use on injuries. The name comfrey derives from the words *con firma*, meaning to unite. The botanical name *Symphytum* comes from *symphyo*, meaning to unite. It was obviously well thought of! It has been grown and used in Britain since at least the Middle Ages. As well as being a medicinal plant it is well known to gardeners as a fertilizer, the leaves being soaked in water for several months and the resulting liquid applied to the soil. The Henry Doubleday Research Association, famous for its pioneering interest in organic gardening, laid great store by the use of comfrey in the garden and as a remedy.

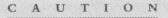

CAUTION

Comfrey leaf and root have been withdrawn from over-the-counter sale recently. There has been evidence in a very small number of cases that where liver disease already exists, excessive consumption has worsened the problem. This has been backed up by experiments on animals where large quantities of comfrey were fed to rats: and this induced liver damage. However, no firm evidence has been produced to show that normal therapeutic doses of the remedy pose any threat and herbal practitioners still have the right to prescribe comfrey at their discretion. Comfrey ointment can be purchased and used by anyone.

Present uses: Using comfrey in the form of an ointment (it is one of the most popular herbal ointments, and easily available from most health/herb shops) is the most widespread practice. It will help speed up the healing of most minor injuries. This is because the constituent called allantion helps

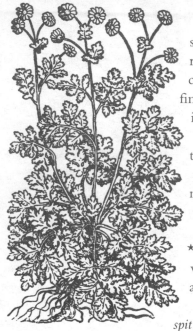

speed up the replication of DNA, after which the rest of the new cell rapidly follows. Thus new cells form, to heal the damaged area. Some people find that the ointment helps as an anti-inflammatory in arthritis problems.

The other beneficial action is the soothing effect that poultices of comfrey have on inflamed skin and ulcers, probably due to the high content of mucilage in the plant. The finely-cut or powdered root is most useful for this purpose.

Combines well with: small amounts of *cayenne and cramp bark, used in an oil as a warming and healing application to 'cold' arthritis and rheumatism problems.

Culpeper says: *'The great comfrey helps those that spit blood, or make bloody urine: the root boiled in water or wine, and the decoction drunk helpeth all inward hurts, bruises and wounds, and the ulcers of the lungs causing the phlegm that oppresseth them to be easily spit forth.'*

CAUTION

Cayenne can be irritating to sensitive mucus membranes and skin. Be careful not to get it in your eyes. Do not apply to broken skin, or to conditions that feel hot and inflamed to start with.

CORIANDER *Coriandrum sativum*
Family: umbelliferae. **Part used:** fruit/seeds and leaves. **Constituents:** volatile oil, tannin. **Action:** aromatic, carminative, stimulant. **Helps to:** aid the digestion, reduce flatulence and colic.
Historical notes: This plant was used by the Greeks and probably brought to Britain by the Romans. The flavour varies depending on the country of origin of the plant, and English coriander is credited with possessing the best flavour. The fresh leaves are increasingly used in cooking for their fine flavour.

Present uses: Make the seeds into a tea to aid the digestion. This remedy is thought to have a stronger action than most of the other aromatics, so keep the strength fairly low. It will also help to promote resistance to the adverse effects of cold weather.

Combines well with: other aromatics if you prefer their taste.

Culpeper says: *'The green herb Coriander being boiled with crumbs of white bread, or barley meal, consumeth and driveth away hot humours, swellings and inflammations and with bean-meal it dissolveth the King's evil, and hard knobs thereof.'*

CORNSILK *Zea mays*

Family: graminaceae. **Part used:** flower pistils (long silky strands found at the end of the cobs). **Constituents:** alkaloid, acids, resins, oil, sugar. **Action:** soothing diuretic. **Helps to:** reduce discomfort in urinary problems

Historical notes: Maize cobs are a familiar part of the diet in Central America, and are credited with some ability to relieve bladder discomfort. When applied as a poultice, the maize grains are considered beneficial to arthritis problems. The remains of the flowers found at the end of the cob are called the cornsilk, and have long been used in America (and Europe since the plant was introduced) for urinary problems.

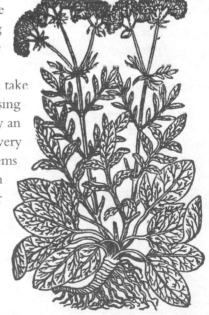

Present uses: Prepare the silk into a tea and take it to help just about any problem causing discomfort in the bladder. It is not specifically an anti-infective remedy, but it does have a very soothing effect and is thus useful for problems such as chills or inflammation not due to an infection. It will help reduce discomfort after an infection has been dealt with by other treatments.

Combines well with: cranberry juice, which should be taken at the same time to reduce the risk of infections developing.

CRAMP BARK
Viburnum opulus

Family: caprifoliaceae. **Part used:** bark.
Constituents: resin, tannin, bitter glycoside:
viburnin (main active constituent). **Action:** antispasmodic, mild astringent.
Helps to: relieve muscle cramp, induce relaxation.

Historical notes: It was considered a valuable enough remedy to be included in the United States *Pharmocopoeia* at one time. The wild variety is the one used medicinally, but a closely related variety remains a popular garden shrub in Britain, and is known as the guelder rose or snowball bush because of its dense clumps of white flowers in the spring. These are followed by red berries, of which Chaucer said, 'picke hem right as they grow and ete hem in', and they 'shal be for your hele'. The berries are in fact very bitter and unpalatable, but do contain a good amount of Vitamin C, which may have been the reason for Chaucer's recommendation.

Present uses: This is the first remedy to consider for problems involving muscle cramps and tension. It is very useful whether the tension results from a physical cause (many painful conditions cause reflex muscle tension, which then adds to the discomfort) or from a psychological cause, such as stress reactions. It is very useful for post-exercise cramps. Use by making a decoction of the bark.

Combines well with: other relaxing remedies such as *passion flower and scullcap, to help reduce reactions to stress. Try this if there is a marked component of muscle-tension in the problem. I have also used cramp bark externally, mixed with *cayenne and comfrey, to make an effective lotion for rheumatism and arthritis.

CAUTION

Passion flower should not be taken in pregnancy.
Cayenne can be irritating to sensitive mucus membranes and skin.
Be careful not to get it in your eyes. Do not apply to broken skin,
or to conditions that feel hot and inflamed to start with.

CUDWEED *Gnaphalium uliginosum*
Family: compositae. **Part used:** leaves and stems. **Constituents:** volatile oil, tannin. **Action:** astringent, anticatarrhal. **Helps to:** soothe sore throats, reduce catarrh.

Present uses: Make into a tea and take to ease sore throats (it has a good effect even in severe problems such as quinsy), laryngitis, head-colds and persistent catarrh (though the cause of this must be tracked down – sometimes it is due to problems in the diet, or to elimination problems, etc.).
Combines well with: peppermint and elderflower, which are also very beneficial for catarrh problems. Use with ★red sage to relieve a sore throat.

C A U T I O N

Do not take red sage in pregnancy.

DAMIANA *Turnera diffusa*
Family: turneraceae. **Part used:** leaves and stem. **Constituents:** volatile oil, bitters, resins, tannins. **Action:** nervine, male and female tonic. **Helps to:** reduce nervous tension, restore sense of vitality.

Historical notes: It has been considered an aphrodisiac in the past, favoured mainly for the treatment of men.

Present uses: Prepared as a tea, damiana is used equally nowadays for its benefit on the nervous and reproductive systems. It is one of the remedies I use most frequently to help problems where depression and anxiety coexist, where a strengthening action rather than either a stimulant or a sedating effect is desirable. Although it has a strong traditional

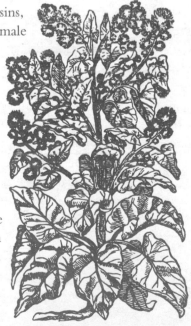

reputation as an aphrodisiac, and particularly as a male tonic, I have never found problems of sexual function to be staightforward enough to be treated successfully with any one remedy. I have found it to be most valuable in treating female reproductive problems, including the emotional instability and tiredness connected with premenstrual syndrome.

Combines well with: wood betony for an effective calming and tonic combination to help stress problems.

DANDELION
Taraxacum officinale

Family: compositae. **Part used:** leaf and root. **Constituents:** *leaf:* flavonoids, minerals, Vitamin C; *root:* glycosides, acids, sugars, minerals, Vitamins A, B, C, D. **Action:** *leaf:* bitter, diuretic; *root:* bitter, cholagogue, gentle laxative. **Helps to:** *leaf:* improve the appetite and digestion, expel excess fluid via the kidneys; *root:* improve the appetite and digestion, ease bowel-motions, stimulate liver functions.

Historical notes: The common name is derived from the French *dent de lion,* meaning lion's teeth, thought to refer to the saw-toothed appearance of the leaves. The same meaning occurs in most other European languages. The botanical name *Taraxacum* comes from the Greek: *taraxos* means disorder and *akos* means remedy - though there is an alternative suggestion that the meaning could be more like 'I have caused pain'!

The young leaves make a pleasant addition to a spring salad, though on maturing they become very bitter. Blanching in the same way as chicory will keep the flavour milder. In Wales the roots and leaves were grated and used in salads.

Dandelion leaf was an ingredient in the herb beers that were popular in the past, and the flowers are used in the famous dandelion wine. A traditional recipe for this is as follows. Take 5.4 litres (1 gallon) of the flowers and pour over them 5.4 litres (1 gallon) of boiling water. Allow to stand for three days, then strain off the liquid and boil it for thirty minutes, adding 1.5kg (3 1/2lb) of sugar, a little sliced fresh root ginger, and the rind of an orange and a lemon. Leave the liquid to stand until tepid, then add yeast to ferment it (a reliable commercial strain of yeast will be available from a brewing shop – follow the directions on the packet) and allow the fermentation to proceed until no more bubbles are given off (a demijohn with a fermentation air-lock will give the most reliable results). Leave for two months before bottling. The flavour has been described as somewhat whiskey-like, and the wine has been considered to have good tonic properties in the past.

Roasted dandelion roots can be used as an alternative to coffee. The commercial product has had the bitterness removed, and has a very mild flavour as a result. The advantage of the drink is that it does not cause the nervous stimulation that ordinary coffee does, so it can be drunk late in the evening with no problems of sleeplessness to follow. The unprocessed dandelion root must be obtained if the medicinal benefit is required.

Present uses: Dandelion leaf is the most effective remedy available for clearing excess fluid from the body. It is ideal for this purpose as many other diuretics, while increasing the loss of fluid, also deplete the body of valuable minerals that are lost at the same time. Dandelion leaves are naturally so rich in minerals that each time a dose is taken, it automatically supplies a good measure of minerals at the same time. To get the beneficial action take a tea of the leaves, dried or fresh, every three hours until the excess fluid has been passed. It is a useful remedy to counteract premenstrual fluid retention.

The root made into a decoction is an ideal stimulant to the appetite, to the function of the stomach and liver, and in a gentle way to the bowel. It is useful in problems such as jaundice and gallbladder disease.

Combines well with: in aiding kidney and liver function, the leaf and root may be useful together for arthritis and rheumatism problems. Mix with clivers and nettles for a good 'blood purifying' combination.

Culpeper says: *'It is of an opening and cleaning quality, and therefore very effectual for the obstructions of the liver, gall, and spleen, and the diseases that arise from them as the jaundice and hypochondriacal passion. It wonderfully openeth the passages of urine, both in young and old.'*

DILL *Anethum graveolens*
Family: umbelliferae. **Part used:** fruit/seed. **Constituents:** volatile oil. **Action:** aromatic, carminative. **Helps to:** improve the digestion, reduce flatulence.

Historical notes: The Greek name for this plant is *anethon*. It was mentioned in the gospel of St Matthew as one of the spices possessed by the Pharisees, along with mint and cummin, and was wrongly thought by English translators to mean aniseed. It was also known to the Greeks and Romans, and has been used in Britain at least since the Middle Ages. Folklore suggests that it was used by witches and magicians in their spells.

Dill is a favourite culinary herb, and imparts a delicious taste to vinegar if the seeds are added a few days before use. In Germany it is used in this way to flavour pickling vinegar, particularly for cucumber pickles. It is also one constituent of the gripe-water formula traditionally used to soothe babies' colic.

Present uses: A tea made from the fruit/seeds is very similar in action to caraway, and is very pleasant to take for digestive disturbances and flatulence. It will help reduce colic and abdominal discomfort.

Combines well with: ginger (the two are used in gripe-water). These two can also be used together in a tea.

Culpeper says: *'The dill being boiled, and drunk, is good to ease swellings and pains; it also stayeth the belly and stomach from casting; and the decoction thereof helpeth women that are troubled with the pains and windiness of the mother. It stayeth the hiccough, being boiled in wine. The seed is of more use than the leaves, and more effectual to digest raw and viscous humours, and is used in medicines that serve to expel wind, and the pains proceeding therefrom. The seed being toasted or fried, and used in oils and plasters, dissolveth imposthumes in the fundament and drieth up all ulcers, especially in the secret parts.'*

Dock
See Yellow Dock

Echinacea
Echinacea angustifolia

Family: compositae. **Part used:** root.
Constituents: volatile oil, alkaloids, acids.
Action: antibacterial, antiviral, immune system stimulant. **Helps to:** support the body's defences against infection.

Historical notes: It was used to treat the life-threatening epidemics of the past, such as typhoid fever.

Present uses: Although we do not have to cope with such severe problems as typhoid any more, echinacea is still the most valuable remedy for the thousands of minor infections we do have to fight off nowadays. Taken as a decoction, the root is the first thing to try if the immune system seems below par. This is useful to build up a person's resistance to infection, and it can be used against respiratory infections, boils, acne (which is due to the

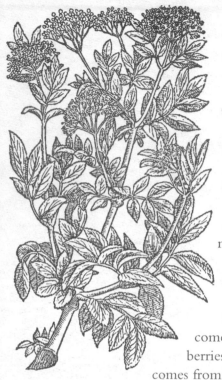

bacteria on the skin feeding on skin secretions), or any viral infections. It will also help against chronic (long-term) infections that might be resistant to antibiotics.

Combines well with: boneset and garlic to help against feverish infections.

E L D E R *Sambucus nigra*
Family: caprifoliaceae. **Part used**: flower and berry. **Constituents**: flavonoids, acids, mucilage, tannins, minerals, volatile oil. **Action**: diaphoretic, diuretic, anticatarrhal. **Helps to**: reduce fevers, reduce catarrh. **Historical notes**: Folklore has it that the English summer starts when the elder comes into flower (June) and ends when the berries are ripe (September). The common name comes from the Anglo-Saxon word *aeld*, meaning fire. The twigs of the elder were easily hollowed out and then blown down in the direction of a fire to help kindle it. Hollow tubes of elderwood have also been used to make musical pipes in various European countries and, similarly, pop-gun toys.

More folklore is attached to elder than to just about any other herb. It used to be a symbol of grief, and it was said to be an elder tree that Judas hanged himself from. Another story held that the tree never grew straight because it was from elderwood that the cross of Jesus was made. Cutting down an elder was thought to bring bad luck, and gypsy people would not use it on their fires. It was featured in pagan myths and associated with magic, and in Russia was thought to give protection against witches and evil forces. In Britain it was carried around as a charm against rheumatism. Sleeping under an elder tree was considered unwise. An infusion of the leaves, which have a distinctly unpleasant smell, has been used by gardeners to protect their crops from insect attacks.

Elderflower water was in the past an official pharmaceutical preparation, used as a mild astringent skin lotion. It was used to keep young ladies' skin from becoming freckled or sunburnt: in the past a suntan was considered undesirable because of its association with lower-class women who had to do outdoor work to make a living. It does help to keep the skin free of blemishes. To make it, fill a crock or pan with elderflowers that you have removed from their stalks, then pour boiling water over them and cover. Allow to cool for a short time, then add three teaspoons of vodka (to act as a preservative) for each 570ml (1 pint) of water used. Leave to stand until cold and then strain and bottle. Apply directly to the skin or add to your bathwater for a relaxing scented soak. Applied to the temples, the water was formerly used to alleviate headaches.

An ointment made from elderflowers was used to treat injured horses during the First World War, and the Blue Cross animal treatment organization made an appeal to the public to collect supplies for its use. The berries have been used as a dye material, for the hair in Roman times and for fabric dyeing up to the present day.

Elderberry wine is a traditional country wine, considered to have similar but weaker properties to those of the flowers. To make the wine, take 2kg (4 1/2lb) of ripe berries (those of the blackest colour), wash and crush them. Then mash 450g (1lb) of bananas and add 450g (1lb) of chopped raisins (both of these are added to improve the flavour and impart more body to the wine). Add all the fruit to 4.5 litres (1 gallon) of water in a large pan. Heat to 85°C for fifteen minutes, then leave to cool. Strain, discard the pulp, and add to the resulting liquid the rind and juice of two oranges and two lemons, and a port wine type yeast and nutrient. Stir in 450g (1lb) of sugar, then pour into a demijohn and seal with a fermentation air-lock. Leave for one week, then add a further 450g (1lb) of sugar. After a second

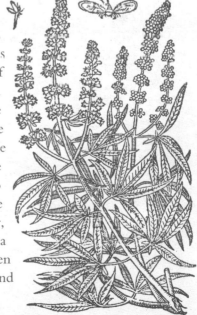

week, add another 450g (1lb) of sugar. Leave until fermentation has finished, then syphon into a clean jar, adding a crushed campden tablet. Store for one or two years, then bottle. If you are patient enough, wait a further six months before drinking!

Present uses: Nowadays the flowers are considered more useful medicinally than the berries. At the first sign of the onset of a feverish cold, elderflowers made into a tea make a very pleasant drink to reduce the discomfort of the symptoms. In chronic catarrhal problems like sinusitis, this can reduce congestion and discomfort.

Combines well with: peppermint, for the traditional combination to help against feverish colds and catarrh problems. Hyssop is a similarly valuable combination.

Culpeper says: *'The juice of the root doth strongly provoke vomiting and purgeth the watery humours of the dropsy. The decoction of the root cureth the biting of a mad dog and also that of the adder; it mollifieth the hardness of the womb, and bringeth down the courses; the berries boiled in wine perform the same effect, and the hair of the head washed therewith is made black.'*

ELECAMPANE *Inula helenium*

Family: compositae. **Part used:** root. **Constituents:** sugars, plant sterols (steroid-like substances), volatile oil. **Action:** expectorant, antitussive (helps reduce a cough) **Helps to:** loosen a tight, dry cough, soothe coughing generally.

Historical notes: It has been known since Roman times, and was used in cooking as well as medicine then. The Greek name is *helenion*, and legends tell of a connection between this plant and Helen of Troy. Eating the roots was thought to help the digestion and the temper. In Britain elecampane has been used since Saxon times, as a remedy and a sweet – the root was candied for this purpose and taken in this form for chest problems and to protect against 'poisonous exhalations and bad air'. The herbalist Gerard recommends it 'against the biting of serpents, it resisteth poison. It is good for them that are bursten and troubled with cramps and convulsions.' In America it was highly thought of as a treatment for skin disease. In France it was used as a flavouring in the drink known as absinthe.

Present uses: This is one of the most reliable remedies for helping in all chest problems, worth trying for infections or allergy problems, acute or chronic. It helps to loosen tight phlegm and soothe the inflamed airways. It is thought to have a certain degree of anti-infective action as well. Make the root into a decoction.

Combines well with: an aromatic chest remedy, such as aniseed, because of elecampane's bitter taste. I also use it with white horehound, which is another rather bitter expectorant. Mix it with *coltsfoot and ginger to loosen tight phlegm, and with *thyme to fight chest infections.

CAUTION

Long-term use of coltsfoot is not recommended.
Do not take thyme in pregnancy.

Culpeper says: *'The roots and herbage beaten and put into new ale or beer, and drunk daily, clear, strengthen and quicken the sight of the eyes exceedingly. The decoction of the roots in wine, or the juice taken therein, killeth and driveth forth all manner of worms in the belly and stomach. The roots being well boiled in vinegar, afterwards beaten and made into an ointment with hog's suet and oil of trotters, is an excellent remedy for the scab or itch.'*

CAUTION

Elecampane has recently been classified as unsuitable for use during pregnancy.

EYEBRIGHT *Euphrasia officinalis*
Family: schrophulariaceae. **Part used:** leaf and stem. **Constituents:** glycosides, volatile oil, astringent substances. **Action:** astringent. **Helps to:** soothe irritated eyes and nasal membranes, soothe sore throats.

Historical notes: The botanical name comes from the Greek word *euphrosyne*, meaning gladness. This is also the word for the linnet, as the story is that this bird was the first creature to discover the benefit of the herb in eye problems, and then gave the knowledge to humans. It has been used for eye diseases since the fourteenth century, and for internal use it has been prepared as tea, wine and ale. One writer explains its use in eye diseases by saying 'the purple and yellow spots and stripes which are upon the flowers of the Eyebright doth very much resemble the diseases of the eye as bloodshot, etc., by which signature it hath been found out that this herb is effectual for the curing of the same'. Traditionally, the expressed juice of the plant, or infusions in milk or water, were used for treatment.

Present uses: This is the most useful remedy for soothing irritated eyes. It does not get rid of infections, but other problems such as irritation due to smoke, air pollution or pollen should respond well. The main action is the astringent effect over the surface of the eye. When I give this remedy, it is in the form of a tincture which is guaranteed to be sterile, diluted with sterile water. If you use it at home you must prepare it as a tea, at the strength of 25g (1oz) of herb to 570ml (1 pint) of water (or scaled down proportionally if you make a smaller amount). Strain it through a very fine filter to ensure you have removed all solid particles, then bathe the eyes as soon as the tea is at body temperature. Prepare the tea freshly each time you use it so there is no risk of introducing an infection into the eyes.

Combines well with: *golden seal, another remedy which is very beneficial for mucus membranes.

C A U T I O N

Golden seal should not be taken in pregnancy, or by people with high blood pressure.

Culpeper says: *'The juice of this herb, taken in white wine, or broth, or dropped into the eyes for several days together, helpeth all the infirmities of them.'*

FENNEL *Foeniculum vulgare*

Family: umbelliferae. **Part used:** fruit and seeds. **Constituents:** volatile oil. **Action.** bitter, aromatic, carminative. **Helps to:** Improve the digestion, reduce flatulence and colic, promote the appetite.

Historical notes: It was cultivated by the Romans for both its edible stems (now grown by gardeners as a separate variety) and its fruits. In Britain it was thought that snakes improved their sight by rubbing their eyes against a fennel plant. People would hang it outside their houses, traditionally on Midsummer's Day to ward off evil spirits, and it had the reputation of protecting against harm from witches and magicians. It was used in the treatment of obesity: 'both the seeds, leaves and root of our Garden Fennel are much used in drinks and broths for those that are grown fat, to abate their unwieldiness and cause them to grow more gaunt and lank' (written in 1650). A drink made from it was also said to confer strength and courage. A sauce flavoured with fennel seeds is a well-known accompaniment to fish dishes. The fleshy lower stem, from the variety known as Florence fennel, is delicious when braised with other vegetables. The flavour is much milder than that of the seeds.

Present uses: Fennel tea is well known for its flavour, similar to aniseed and ★liquorice. It is useful for people with a reduced appetite, particularly when this is associated with flatulence and discomfort.

C A U T I O N

Do not take liquorice in pregnancy.

Culpeper says: *'Fennel is good to break wind, provoke urine and ease the pains of, as well as break, the stone. The leaves and seed boiled in barley water, and drunk, are good to increase milk, and make it more wholesome. The leaves, or rather seed, boiled in water, will stay the hiccoughs and take away the loathing which often happens to the stomach of sick and feverish persons.'*

FENUGREEK
Trigonella foenum-graecum

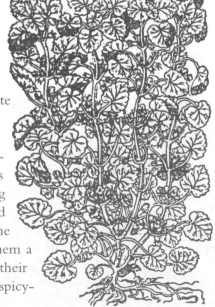

Family: leguminosae. **Part used:** seeds.
Constituents: volatile oil, mucilage, bitters, alkaloids, saponins. **Action:** aromatic, carminative, expectorant, laxative. **Helps to:** improve the appetite and digestion, calm flatulence, reduce menopause symptoms.

Historical notes: The name *foenum-graecum* means 'Greek hay', and the seeds have been used in medicine and cooking since the time of the Greeks and Romans. One technique was to soak the seeds in water, strain them and leave them a few days to sprout, thus maximizing their nutritional content. This would make a spicy-tasting addition to any modern-day salad. For their medicinal benefit, the seeds would be left soaking in water until they formed a mucilaginous consistency, very soothing to the digestive system. The same preparation was also used externally as a poultice to soothe inflamed wounds and ulcers.

Present uses: These seeds are familiar as curry spices and are well known for the pungent scent they create in shops selling spices. They can be taken as a tea to help the appetite and digestion; if soaked overnight in water, the seeds are useful as a gentle, non-griping laxative. When crushed and soaked in hot water, they are used as a poultice on inflamed skin. The steroid-like actions of the remedy are due to the saponins in the seeds. They seem to help women who are having problems because of low oestrogen levels and can be very helpful at the time of the menopause, taken as a tea. The saponins as well as the mucilage are the active constituents when the remedy is used externally as a poultice.

Combines well with: powdered linseed or marshmallow which, when mixed with fenugreek, may make a better consistency for a poultice. *Red sage helps reduce hot flushes in the menopause and can be taken with fenugreek for this problem.

CAUTION

Do not take red sage in pregnancy.

Culpeper says: *'The decoction or broth of the seed, drunk with a little vinegar, expelleth and purgeth all superfluous humours which cleave to the bowels; the same decoction, first made with dates, and afterwards formed into a syrup with honey, mundifieth and cleanseth the breast, chest and lungs, and may be taken with success for any grief attendant thereon.'*

FEVERFEW *Tanacetum parthenium*

Family: compositae. **Part used:** leaf. **Constituents:** volatile oil. **Action:** anti-inflammatory, preventative against migraines. **Helps to:** reduce symptoms of rheumatic and arthritic problems, reduce frequency and severity of most migraine headaches.

Historical notes: This plant was well known in country gardens, being very attractive and easy to grow. It seeds itself readily; if you plant one or two, the following year you will have a dozen. It has a very characteristic pungent, bitter smell rather like tansy, and was planted around doorways to purify the atmosphere. Most people assume the name is connected with the plant's use against feverish conditions, but it is more likely to have originated because of the appearance of the leaves, which are very delicately divided and lacy (feathery – hence the word derived from 'featherfew').

Present uses: Feverfew is most useful in the treatment of arthritis and rheumatism, and also migraines. It has been researched thoroughly in the last few years, and has been found to prevent in part the inflammatory changes that characterize arthritis. This action was discovered during a trial of feverfew on migraine sufferers, when a significant number of them reported that as well as their migraines improving, their arthritis was better too! It seems that about 70 per cent of migraines respond well to feverfew, particularly if they are connected with a feeling of cold, where a warming application would be soothing.

The best way to take the remedy is to obtain a plant and pick about two mature-sized leaves to eat every day. They have a very bitter taste and may be more palatable put into a sandwich – you will still get the benefit of them like this. Unfortunately, the plant is herbaceous and dies off in the winter, so at this time of year there is no alternative but to buy the dried herb to make into a tea, or to take tablets or capsules.

Combines well with: *celery seeds to help arthritis and rheumatism problems.

C A U T I O N

Feverfew is unsuitable for use in pregnancy.
Do not take celery seeds in pregnancy.

Culpeper says: *'It is effectual in removing all pains of the head arising from a cold, the herb being bruised or applied to the crown thereof; used in the same manner, it is likewise good for the swimming or giddiness of the head. A decoction of the flowers in wine, with a little nutmeg or mace therein, drunk several times a day is an approved provocative of women's courses, and to sit over the hot fumes of the decoction of the herb, made in water or wine will prove equally serviceable.'*

FRIAR'S BALSAM SEE BENZOIN

GARLIC *Allium sativa*

Family: liliaceae. **Part used:** bulb – made up of several cloves. **Constituents:** sulphur-containing substances, vitamins, flavonoids, proteins, oils. **Action:** antimicrobial, anti-inflammatory, lowers blood cholesterol levels, lowers blood pressure. **Helps to:** improve the condition of the circulatory system, fight off infections – particularly head-colds, sore throats and chest infections.

Historical notes: The earliest mention of the cultivation and use of garlic, in medicine and cooking, goes back to 1550 BC, to the ancient Egyptians. It has been prized in Mediterranean countries for its flavour ever since, but the objectionable nature of its smell was also referred to by some authors. Its name is from the Anglo-Saxon *gar* (spear) and *lac* (plant), describing the long narrow shape of the leaves.

Garlic was used a good deal in the First World War for its antimicrobial properties – the juice was squeezed onto dressings which were then applied to wounds to reduce the risk of infection. A popular home remedy for chest infections was made by mixing garlic juice with honey and vinegar. This mixture was taken by mouth, though rubbing applications made by soaking garlic in oil or lard were also used.

Present uses: Modern research has more than justified the reputation of garlic throughout the ages. Great benefits to the circulatory and respiratory systems can be gained through the regular consumption of either the fresh, raw clove (not many people are enthusiastic about this) or tablets and capsules containing active extracts of the plant. The sulphur-containing constituents are thought to be responsible for most of the benefits to the circulation. Clinical tests have shown that the regular use of garlic for several months can result in a lowering of cholesterol levels in the blood and the lowering of high blood pressure. The tendency towards the formation of harmful clots in damaged blood vessels is reduced, and the blood is more likely to stay 'thin'. Trials on people who have had an initial heart-attack have shown that if they take garlic the risk of a second one is significantly reduced.

Garlic is useful in head-colds, sinusitis, sore throats and chest infections because it possesses antiviral as well as antibacterial actions. The pungent-smelling active ingredients become concentrated in the lungs, because this is the body's channel of elimination for them. It means unfortunately that

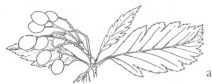

the smell of garlic on the breath cannot be avoided. You might think it has lingered from when you swallowed it, but it is actually because the body is getting rid of it through the membranes lining the lungs. It also permeates through the skin – both in and out – to some extent (if you rub garlic on the soles of your feet you will eventually smell it on your breath).

Many people ask me if the garlic they use in cooking will have this medicinal benefit. Unfortunately, most of the active ingredients are broken down in the process of cooking, as the change in smell from pungent to mellow indicates. To get the full benefit you need to take it raw.

Garlic is easy to grow in Britain. The best results are obtained when the planting is done in the autumn and the bulbs are harvested the following summer. A complete bulb can be broken up into separate cloves, each of which should be planted the same way as onion sets. Bury the clove in the soil with just the top showing above soil level, with about 10cm (4in) between the cloves and 45cm (18in) between rows.

Press the soil firmly around each clove to prevent birds or mice pulling them up. Each clove will produce a whole bulb with up to fifteen new cloves. It is always cultivated rather than wild garlic that is used for its medicinal properties.

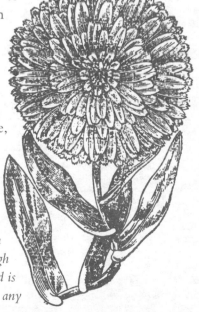

Combines well with: honey – the traditional way of taking garlic which is quite palatable, and soothing for a sore throat. Take echinacea as well for increased effectiveness against infections.

Culpeper says: *'It provoketh urine and women's courses and helpeth the bitings of mad dogs and other venomous creatures. It killeth worms in children, cutteth and bringeth forth tough phlegm, purgeth the head, helpeth the lethargy and is a good preservative against, and a remedy for, any*

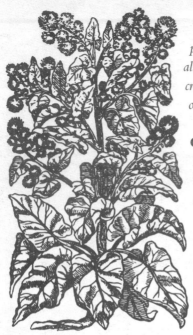

plague sore or foul ulcer. It is also exceeding good in all hydropic diseases, the jaundice, falling sickness, cramps, convulsions, the piles or haemorrhoids, and other cold diseases.'

GENTIAN *Gentiana lutea*

Family: gentianaceae. **Part used:** root. **Constituents:** bitters, sugars, acids, volatile oil. **Action:** bitter tonic, digestive stimulant. **Helps to:** improve the appetite and digestion.

Historical notes: There are several different species of gentians, and it is only the yellow gentian that is used medicinally. It grows wild in Mediterranean countries and can be cultivated quite successfully in Britain. The bitter taste of the root is unmistakeable even in very dilute preparations, and it has been used for this property in brewing and medicine for hundreds of years. It is still prescribed by modern doctors for the problems of convalescence, to help restore the appetite.

Present uses: Yellow gentian can be taken as a tea, made by grating or grinding the root and using only about one eighth of a teaspoon to a cup of boiling water. If this tastes too bitter, just dilute it more until an acceptable strength is achieved (but remember it does have to taste bitter to some extent for you to get the benefit from it). If this drink is sipped slowly about half an hour before meals, it will improve the appetite and efficiency of the digestion. It is useful after debilitating infections such as influenza, when it can take some people weeks to feel normal again. It will also help those who have problems with a generally sluggish digestive function.

Combines well with: one of the aromatic carminative remedies like caraway, to make it more palatable, but don't try to disguise the bitter taste completely.

Culpeper says: *'The powder of the dried root helps the biting of venomous beasts, opens the obstructions of the liver, and restoreth lost appetite. Steeped in wine and* *drunk, it refresheth those that are weary with travelling, it helps stitches and griping pains in the side, and is an excellent remedy for those that are bruised by falls.'*

C A U T I O N

Gentian should not be taken by people who have gastric or duodenal ulcers.

GINGER *Zingiberis officinalis*

Family: zingiberaceae. **Part used:** root (botanically a rhizome). **Constituents:** volatile oil, resin, starch, protein, fats. **Action:** aromatic, carminative, anti-emetic, circulatory stimulant, expectorant. **Helps to:** improve the digestion, and reduce flatulence and colic, reduce motion sickness, reduce susceptibility to illness caused by cold weather.

Historical notes: Ginger has been known in the East since ancient times and was taken to America in the sixteenth century. The West Indies now grow the largest crop worldwide, though Africa and the Far East also export it. It used to be available only in dried form in Britain, but with the growth in popularity of Asian food the fresh root is now seen much more often in greengrocers' shops. Candied ginger is made by soaking the scalded young green roots in a succession of progressively stronger sugar syrups. In the West Indies the discarded syrups were used as a base for a fermented drink. The dried root differs from the fresh in that it is usually less aromatic, due to the loss of some of the oil, but it is more pungent because of the formation of new substances during the drying process. It has been traditionally used to help the digestion. The herbalist Gerard describes it as 'right good with meat in sauces or otherwise in conditures; for it is of an heating and digesting qualitie'.

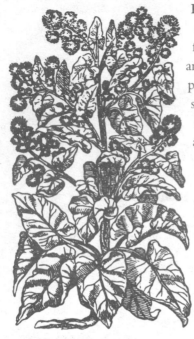

Present uses: If a warming remedy is required, ginger is the most reliable. I use it far more than I do cayenne, as it is less fierce and irritating, and more aromatic. For any problem aggravated by the cold weather, such as arthritis (there may be a specific anti-inflammatory action that ginger has, in addition to the benefit of the warming effect) or bronchitis, it is most helpful. Also, the classic cold weather problem of chilblains will be helped if ginger is taken internally or used in a footbath.

The aromatic properties make it a useful remedy for the digestion, to promote activity in a sluggish stomach or liver and to reduce discomfort due to flatulence or colic. A recently discovered benefit is its effectiveness against motion sickness, without the disadvantage of drowsiness that most of the orthodox drugs for this involve. There are several ways of taking ginger. The dried powdered root is still the most easily-available form and can be added to hot drinks (because of the pungency, you will use it in much smaller amounts than most other remedies: try a pinch of the powder to start with). If the fresh root is available you can slice it very finely and make a tea using about a quarter of a teaspoonful. For external use, make a footbath by adding the tea to pleasantly warm water and immerse your feet for about ten minutes (if the skin on your feet is broken the ginger might sting, so start with a very dilute tea, about the same strength as suggested for the drinks). Crystallized ginger is an enjoyable sweet, and convenient for travellers prone to motion sickness to take.

Combines well with: other cough remedies such as *elecampane in cases of chest infections, and with other aromatics such as caraway for the digestion.

> ## CAUTION
> ·······························
> *Do not take elecampane in pregnancy.*

GINSENG *Panax ginseng*

Family: araliaceae. **Part used:** root. **Constituents:** glycosides, saponins, volatile oil, sugars, starch. **Action:** stimulant, tonic for nervous system. **Helps to:** improve the ability to cope with stress and work. **Historical notes:** In China this was considered to be almost a cure-all plant, used to help the sick recover and the healthy to achieve more vitality. It grows wild in the Far East and North America, and American supplies have been imported into China since the eighteenth century to meet the huge demand for it. The profits obtained were enormous; as a result of this, wild specimens in America have now become rare, and cultivation and export are strictly controlled to avoid the plant becoming extinct. It was used traditionally by native Americans, who only collected those plants that bore mature fruits. These were planted as the roots were gathered, thus ensuring the continuation of the species.

Present uses: Ginseng became popular a few years ago when it gained a reputation as an aphrodisiac. There is no firm evidence to support this, but it does seem to help people cope better with stress and infections. It has a beneficial action on the immune system, the circulation and the nervous system. The outcome of this is that it helps improve physical and mental performance in demanding situations, such as during examinations or when working long hours. It is helpful during convalescence, to restore the appetite and stamina. It is believed in China that ginseng helps to delay the ageing process and to maintain a healthy vigour into old age. It is available in root form to take as a decoction, or as tablets or capsules. The recommended dose is 0.6-2g daily (don't go above this).

CAUTION

Ginseng should not be taken continuously for more than one month. Leave a period of one to two months before taking it again. It should not be taken during pregnancy or by people with high blood pressure. Do not take other stimulants, including coffee, while taking ginseng.

GOLDEN ROD *Solidago virgaurea*

Family: compositae. **Part used:** leaf and stem. **Constituents:** saponins, flavonoids, astringents. **Action:** anticatarrhal, diuretic, diaphoretic. **Helps to:** reduce catarrh, aid recovery from cystitis.

Historical notes: Golden rod has been used for serious fever-causing diseases because of its diaphoretic and diuretic properties. It had a reputation for helping the passing of kidney stones, but the large sizes claimed for these

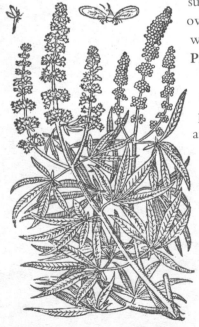

suggest that the anecdotes about it may have been overenthusiastic. Externally it was used on wounds and ulcers for its astringent properties.

Present uses: The main condition for which I use this herb is chronic catarrh. This is not necessarily connected with an infection: some people have problems with nasal congestion and sinusitis all year round. Golden rod taken as a tea is well worth trying to alleviate this, although of course it may not address the cause of the problem.

Combines well with: marsh cudweed: the combination gives better results than either remedy used separately. A range of other remedies may also be needed to deal with the underlying causes of the problem.

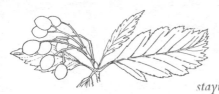

Culpeper says: '*The decoction of the herb, either green or dry, or the distilled water thereof, is very effectual for inward bruises, likewise for staying the floodings of the body, as fluxes of humours, bloody fluxes, and the immoderate menses of women.*'

GOLDEN SEAL *Hydrastis canadensis*

Family: ranunculaceae. **Part used:** root. **Constituents:** alkaloids, resins, acids, starch, volatile oil. **Action:** antimicrobial, cholagogue, laxative, anticatarrhal. **Helps to:** stimulate the digestion, reduce catarrh, improve resistance to infections.

Historical notes: The plant is a native of North America, and European settlers learnt of its medicinal value from the native Americans. In the late nineteenth century its popularity grew; as more was taken from the wild and its habitat destroyed, it became rare and ever more expensive. It was used by the native Americans for digestive problems, applied externally to wounds and ulcers and used to bathe the eyes. In the North American physiomedical tradition it was considered a sovereign remedy for any problem concerning mucus membranes, and used for digestive and respiratory problems.

Present uses: For digestive problems where liver or gallbladder function is involved, golden seal is an excellent remedy. It helps as a laxative if necessary, but I haven't found this to be a strong action: you can still take it even if you don't actually need a laxative effect. It is also very useful for head-colds, sore throats and catarrh problems generally. Golden seal is one of the few remedies thought to help the condition of the veins, and so is worth taking for problems like varicose veins and fluid retention due to incompetent veins. The root should be made into a decoction, or if the powdered form is available this can be prepared as a tea. You will need this remedy in small amounts only - try about one eighth to one quarter of a teaspoonful to make each dose. These preparations make very good local treatments, such as a gargle for sore throats and a lotion with which to bathe the eyes. If you intend to make the eye lotion, remember that it must be filtered to remove all particles of the powder or solid herb, and that you must make a fresh preparation from boiling water to ensure that it is sterile. The eye lotion should be only about one quarter of the strength of the normal preparation - the easiest way to make this is to dilute the tea with sterile water.

Combines well with: any of the aromatic remedies used to help the digestion, or with peppermint and elderflower to help catarrh problems. It is used with eyebright in eye lotions.

C A U T I O N

Golden seal should not be taken in pregnancy, or by people who have high blood pressure.

GROUND IVY *Glechoma hederacea*
Family: labiateae. **Part used:** leaf and stem. **Constituents:** bitters, tannins, volatile oil. **Action:** anticatarrhal, expectorant, diuretic. **Helps to:** reduce nasal and throat catarrh, reduce catarrh-induced tinnitus (ringing in the ears).

Historical notes: The common name for this plant comes from the resemblance of its leaves to the true ivy, though they are much smaller. It was used by the Saxons as an addition to beer, to help give a bitter flavour and preserve the drink (both properties are due to the bitters in the plant). It has a long reputation for treating respiratory disease and for being a good blood purifier.

Culpeper says: '... *if you put to the decoction some honey, ... it is excellent good to gargle any sore mouth or throat, and to wash the sores and ulcers ... it helpeth the itch, scabs, wheals, and other breakings out, in any part of the body.*'

Present uses: The bitters and tannins make ground ivy a useful remedy for catarrhal problems, and possibly its other eliminative actions also contribute to the benefit. Take it as a tea, at the standard strength, to help reduce catarrh and clear phlegm from the chest. This benefit can also reduce the problem of ringing noises and pressure sensations in the ears, which are generally aggravated by catarrh.

Combines well with: boneset and hyssop or elderflower for a good anticatarrhal remedy.

HAWTHORN

Crataegus oxyacantha, platyphyllos or cordata species

Family: rosaceae. **Part used:** berries, leaves and flowers. **Constituents:** tannins, saponins, flavonoids, acids (including Vitamin C: ascorbic acid).

Action: heart tonic, reduces high blood pressure. **Helps to:** strengthen the heartbeat without affecting the rate, normalize a high blood pressure, possibly improve the condition of diseased arteries.

Historical notes: The botanical name comes from the Greek words *kratos*, which means hard and describes the character of the wood of this tree, *andoxus* and *akantha*, meaning sharp thorn. The common name means a hedge thorn, which tells us that the tree was used in the past to indicate the boundaries between different pieces of land. Christian folklore says that the hawthorn was the tree from which Christ's crown of thorns was made, and it was considered sacred as a result. The young, tender leaves used to be eaten; they had the nickname of 'bread and butter' (I can't say I notice much similarity in the tastes). The berries of various hawthorn species are used to make preserves.

Present uses: If there is one remedy universally applicable to *heart problems, it is hawthorn. I generally use the berries, but the flowers are valuable as well. It helps as a steady support for the functioning of the heart and blood vessels, improving the efficiency of the circulation, reducing high blood pressure and bringing the further benefits of this to the whole constitution. The fresh or dried berries can be taken as a tea: the dose is half a teaspoon of the dried, crushed berries or twice that of the fresh berries.

Combines well with: yarrow and limeflowers for an effective combination against high blood pressure, and with *motherwort to help with heart problems.

Culpeper says: *'The seeds, bruised and boiled in wine, will give instant relief to the tormenting pains of the body. If cloths and sponges are wet in the distilled water, and applied to any place wherein thorns, splinters, &etc are lodged, it will certainly draw them forth.'*

CAUTION

Seek professional help immediately if heart problems are suspected. Hawthorn should not be used in place of a professional diagnosis. Do not take motherwort in the first eight months of pregnancy.

Hops *Humulus lupulus*

Family: cannabinaceae. **Part used:** strobile (fruiting body). **Constituents:** resinous bitters, volatile oil, flavonoids. **Action:** aromatic bitter, sedative, antispasmodic. **Helps to:** improve the appetite, reduce flatulence and colic, induce relaxation and sleep.

Historical notes: In Roman times the plant was cultivated for its young shoots, which were eaten as a vegetable. It grows wild in the south of England and is cultivated on a large scale to supply the brewing industry. The name comes from the Anglo-Saxon word *hoppan*, which means to climb. In Saxon times fermented drinks were made from malt and flavoured with various bitter and aromatic herbs such as wormwood and yarrow, and hops were not used until the sixteenth century. After this time the distinction between 'ale' (the earlier drink made without hops) and 'beer' (meaning bitter) was made. Hops were originally added as a preservative, so that the drink could be kept fresher-tasting and transported further. There was some controversy about this development: in the reign of Henry VIII a petition was brought to Parliament condemning the hop as 'a wicked weed that would spoil the taste of the drink and endanger the people'. There was a belief that hops could cause 'melancholy', similar to today's cautions about its use.

Nowadays practically all hop cultivation in Britain is in the counties of Kent and Herefordshire. After the plant flowers (male and female flowers occur on separate plants) the female plants develop the papery cone-like strobiles that are rich in a powdery resin. This is chiefly what gives the bitter properties, and the strobiles are carefully collected and dried in a way that conserves the resin and oils. The stimulating action that bitters have on the digestion has led to the custom of taking bitter drinks like beer before meals. The other main property of hops, the relaxing action, has been utilized in the making of pillows stuffed with hops as a treatment for insomnia.

Present uses: As in the past, the two uses of hops relate to their bitterness and their sedative properties. Taken as a drink (a moderate amount of beer is the obvious one, or an infusion of the strobiles for people who want to avoid alcohol) about half an hour before eating, the appetite will be sharpened and the digestion improved. The volatile oil also helps benefit the digestion, allaying flatulence and colic. The calming effect is useful at night for people who have problems sleeping. Some patent herbal preparations to help with relaxation contain hops, and are available in tea mixtures and tablet form.

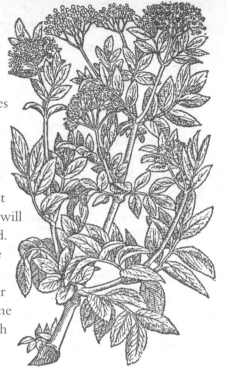

Combines well with: other relaxing remedies such as chamomile to help both digestion and nerves, as they are more palatable than hops by themselves.

Culpeper says: *'In cleansing the blood, they help to cure the French disease, and all manner of scabs, itch, and other breakings-out of the body; also tetters, ringworms, and spreading sores, the morphew and all discolourings of the skin.'*

C A U T I O N

Because of the sedative properties of hops, they should not be taken by people who have problems with depression.

HORSETAIL *Equisetum arvense*
Family: equisetaceae. **Part used:** aerial parts (different botanically from most other plants because, as a very primitive plant, it does not have true

leaves). **Constituents:** flavonoids, alkaloids, minerals – mainly silicates. **Action:** diuretic, haemostatic. **Helps to:** reduce discomfort in bladder inflammation, promote the healing of wounds and external ulcers.

Historical notes: This plant is so named because of its appearance: it is thought to resemble a horse's tail, though to me it looks more like a bottle-brush. It is well known to gardeners as a weed that is virtually impossible to get rid of; the stems are very brittle and always snap off leaving part of the plant in the soil. There is a noticeable gritty feel to the stems, due to their high silicate content. Three hundred million years ago very similar plants grew to enormous sizes and formed much of the material that was later fossilized as coal. Horsetail is more closely related to ferns than to flowering plants. It was eaten as a vegetable by those Romans who could afford nothing else, but it was not highly praised. Northern European farmers sometimes used it for cattle-fodder, but it tended to wear down the animals' teeth. It has been used as an abrasive for cleaning metal and wood because of the silicates it contains, and has been called 'scouring rushes' and 'pewterwort'. It had a great reputation as a remedy to stop blood flow and to heal wounds and ulcers when applied externally.

Present uses: It is a most effective soothing remedy for bladder and prostate gland problems. Its function is not to get rid of an infection, so it must be used with other remedies to achieve this, but it has a very soothing effect on the discomfort caused by infections, chills or other sources of irritation. It has been used to treat bed-wetting in children, but this is rarely a straightforward physical problem so success cannot be guaranteed.

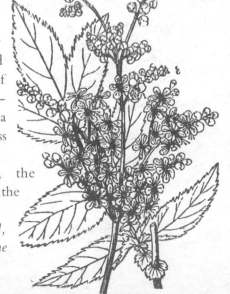

Combines well with: *bearberry, the most reliable anti-infective remedy for the urinary tract.

Culpeper says: *'It stays fluxes of every kind, either in men or women; suppresses the* *evacuation of blood through the urinary passages, and healeth not only the inward ulcers and excoriation of the entrails, bladder, &c. but all other sorts of foul, moist and running ulcers, and quickly healeth green wounds.'*

C A U T I O N

Horsetail should not be taken by people with heart or kidney problems. Bearberry should not be taken in pregnancy or by people with kidney problems

HYSSOP *Hyssopus officinalis*
Family: labiatae. **Part used:** leaves and flowers. **Constituents:** volatile oil, flavonoids. **Action:** expectorant, diaphoretic, carminative. **Helps to:** ease a feverish head-cold, soothe a cough, improve the digestion.

Historical notes: Hyssop has been known since biblical times, but there is some dispute as to whether the plant mentioned numerous times in the Bible is the one we know as hyssop today. It has been used for respiratory problems for hundreds of years. It also had a reputation for easing rheumatism, and was used internally and as a lotion for this. The oil of the plant is used in perfumery and it is one of the ingredients in Chartreuse liqueur.

Present uses: A tea made of hyssop is an excellent drink to take at the onset of head-colds and 'flu. It helps regulate a high temperature and is useful to ease catarrh. Take it regularly to ease chronic catarrh, although other remedies will also be required to treat the causes of this. It helps with chest infections too, and is worth using to ease coughs. Although less used now than in the past for digestive problems, it will help reduce flatulence and colic. It has useful relaxing properties, and is considered specific for the type of minor epilepsy known as 'petit mal'.

Combines well with: boneset to treat a feverish cold or 'flu, and with elderflower and peppermint for long-term catarrh. Take hyssop with one of the aromatic carminatives like caraway or cardamom for digestive problems.

Culpeper says: *'Being boiled in wine, it is good to wash inflammations, and taketh away the black and blue spots, and marks proceeding from blows, bruises or falls, if applied with warm water. It is a good remedy for the stinging of serpents; the head being anointed with the oil thereof, it killeth the lice and allayeth the itchings of the same.'*

Lavender
Lavandula officinalis

Family: labiatae. **Part used:** flowers. **Constituents:** volatile oil. **Action:** aromatic, carminative, nervine. **Helps to:** improve the digestion, reduce flatulence and colic, ease nervous tension.

Historical notes: This favourite cottage garden plant has been prized for its scent since Elizabethan times. It is a native of the Mediterranean and was used by the Romans for scent and medicine - its use in the bath accounts for its name, as *lavare* is the Latin word for 'to wash'. It was mentioned in the Bible as the much-valued 'Spikenard', and spike lavender is another name for it. There are now many varieties for the gardener to choose from and many grades of oil are extracted from the flowers, the quality depending on the conditions in which they have been grown. Lavender was one of the herbs thought to give protection from the plague in the Middle Ages, and there are many customs and folklore rituals in which it figures. It was taken to the New World by the Pilgrim Fathers in the seventeenth century. In most rural houses where it was grown the flowers would be picked and dried, to be used in toiletries, medicine or perfumery. Lavender bags were used to scent linen and clothes in storage.

As a medicine, lavender was thought to help against the bites of snakes and mad dogs, and was taken to relieve pain and reduce stress and tension problems. Externally it was used as a lotion or poultice for painful problems like neuralgia, headaches and toothache. The oil has been used on skin injuries like burns and ulcers, and modern research is confirming its value.

The lavender industry in Britain is centred around south-east England and East Anglia. Most of the crop goes to prepare oil of lavender, used in perfumery.

Present uses: It may seem strange to use what we think of exclusively as a perfume for medicinal purposes, but lavender makes a good remedy for the digestion and an excellent one for easing nervous tension. The taste is not unpleasant (being largely influenced by the sense of smell) when you have got used to the idea of it. Make a tea of the flowers, ideally picked soon after they have opened. A pleasant way to get the relaxing benefit at night is to make a sachet containing dried lavender and hops and keep it on your pillow. Tincture of lavender is very helpful for drying up cold sores. A lotion of lavender makes a good external application for headaches, and oil of lavender is a very useful first-aid remedy for damaged skin. Get some advice when you buy this, as there is a great deal of variation in the quality.

Combines well with: carminatives such as caraway, or with other relaxing remedies such as *passion flower and wood betony for stress problems or headaches. The infused oil can be mixed with rosemary oil to make a relaxing and restorative massage oil, or with peppermint oil as a lotion to apply to the temples to treat headaches.

Culpeper says: *'Lavender is of special use for pains in the head and brain that do proceed of a cold cause, as the apoplexy, falling sickness, the drowsy or sluggish* *malady, cramps, convulsions, palsies and often faintings. It strengtheneth the stomach and freeth the liver and spleen from obstructions, and provoketh women's courses.'*

C A U T I O N

Do not take passion flower during pregnancy.

LEMON BALM *Melissa officinalis*

Family: labiatae. **Part used:** leaf and stem. **Constituents:** volatile oil, bitters, tannins. **Action:** carminative, nervine. **Helps to:** improve the digestion, calm nervous indigestion, ease nervous tension.

Historical notes: The name balm is a short form of balsam, meaning sweet-smelling. Lemon balm has always been prized for its action against nervous problems, and the advice of the London Dispensary of 1696 is that 'an essence of Balm, given in Canary wine, every morning will renew youth, strengthen the brain, relieve languishing nature and prevent baldness'. It was used as a wound application, to staunch bleeding and help healing. The dried leaves have been an ingredient of pot-pourri mixtures because of their delicious scent.

Present uses: Lemon balm is so easily grown in the garden that the best way to use it is to make a tea of the fresh leaves. These have a lovely lemon fragrance and can be used as a refreshing alternative to ordinary tea in the summer. The specific benefits are the easing of digestive and stress problems, with indigestion due to nervous tension the classic indication.

Combines well with: other relaxing remedies like *passion flower and wood betony to improve their flavour, and it is a pleasant enough drink to take by itself.

Culpeper says: *'Let a syrup be made with the juice of it and sugar, be kept in every gentlewoman's house, to relieve the weak stomachs and sick bodies of their poor and sickly neighbours, as also the herb kept dry in the house, so that, with other convenient simples, you may make it into an electuary with honey, according as the disease is.'*

C A U T I O N

Do not take passion flower during pregnancy

LIMEFLOWERS

Tilia cordata or platyphyllos

Family: tiliaceae. **Part used:** flowers and attached bract. **Constituents:** volatile oil, mucilage, tannins, saponins, flavonoids. **Action:** diaphoretic, relaxing. **Helps to:** reduce high blood pressure, reduce nervous tension, reduce fevers, improve the circulation.

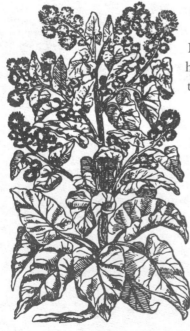

Historical notes: Limeflowers used to be a household remedy for hysteria, nervous tension and indigestion. They were used in France for the tea known as *tilleul*, and are mentioned as such in Proust's novel about his childhood: 'A la Recherche du Temps Perdu' ('Remembrance of Times Past'). The wood of the tree is valued by wood-carvers and turners, and charcoal from the wood has been used to treat flatulence. The leaves and flowers are very mucilaginous and have been used to get a good consistency for poultices.

Present uses: Limeflower tea (also known as linden) makes a very pleasant drink as an alternative to ordinary tea. Its specific medical benefits include improvements to the circulation, the reduction of high blood pressure and reduction of nervous tension generally (it makes a useful late-night drink to help improve sleeping). It is one of the remedies most suited to children and if a baby is too young to take it by mouth the tea can be added to the bathwater to help the chance of a good night's sleep. It is a useful drink to take for head-colds, as it helps against fevers and catarrh. I have used it successfully in cases of eczema for its relaxing and circulatory properties.

Combines well with: yarrow to help high blood pressure and eczema. Mix it with chamomile to have a calming effect or with catmint to help reduce feverishness in children.

Culpeper says: *'The flowers of the linden tree are good against falling sickness; so likewise is the distilled water of the bark; and is also serviceable against those fretting humours which occasion the bloody flux, and griping in the guts.'*

LIQUORICE *Glycyrrhiza glabra*

Family: leguminosae. **Part used:** root. **Constituents:** glycosides, saponins, flavonoids, bitters, volatile oil, tannins, oestrogen-related substances. **Action:** expectorant, anti-arthritic, laxative, demulcent. **Helps to:** loosen tight phlegm, reduce inflammation in rheumatism and arthritis, improve bowel function, protect the sites of gastric and duodenal ulcers against stomach acid.

Historical notes: The first recorded use of liquorice was in the third century BC in the Near East. It was known to the Greeks and Romans, and the name comes from Greek words meaning sweet root. It was used in Britain by the thirteenth century.

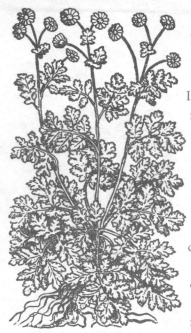

Present uses: Liquorice makes a palatable addition to any cough mixture, helping to loosen tight phlegm and reduce discomfort in the lungs. It is also valuable in the treatment of arthritis and rheumatism. Several of the constituents combine to give it a useful anti-inflammatory action that can help reduce pain and swelling in arthritic joints. For problems of overacidity in the stomach, liquorice has a valuable protective action. It will cut down on the risk of damage to the lining of the stomach, which otherwise could lead to the development of ulcers. It helps form a protective coating of mucus over the site of already existing ulcers, so that they can heal more easily, free from the adverse effects of further exposure to stomach acid.

You can buy pure liquorice juice sticks at many herb/health shops. These are beneficial to chew on instead of eating sweets, and you will get some of the therapeutic effects this way. Otherwise you can make the root into a tea.

Combines well with: other cough remedies like *elecampane and white horehound for a more palatable combination. For the digestion, try marshmallow root, meadowsweet and liquorice. This is particularly useful for problems of overacidity.

Culpeper says: *'Liquorice boiled in clear water with some maiden-hair and figs, it maketh a good drink for such as are troubled with a dry cough, hoarseness, wheezing or shortness of breath, and for all complaints of the breast and lungs, phthisic or consumptions, caused by the distillation of salt humours on them.'*

C A U T I O N

Do not take liquorice or elecampane in pregnancy.
Occasionally it may cause swelling in the ankles.

MARIGOLD *Calendula officinalis*

Family: compositae. **Part used:** flowers. **Constituents:** volatile oil, saponins, resin, bitters. **Action:** aromatic, antispasmodic, diaphoretic, haemostatic, antiseptic. **Helps to:** heal stomach and duodenal ulcers, promote skin healing, clear fungal infections, prevent deterioration in varicose veins.

Historical notes: Although the Latin name of the marigold refers to the fact that it is reputed to be in flower on the calends (or first day) of each month, most gardeners will know that it usually flowers between May and October. The origin of the English name may date back to Anglo-Saxon times, although some think that it is named after the Virgin Mary. No one who has ever seen the deep orange, golden flower can doubt where the latter part of the name came from.

There are several types of marigold grown in gardens today. Make sure you have the traditional English pot marigold if you want to use it medicinally – the African and French types are quite different and don't have any therapeutic properties.

Present uses: This is one of the best-known remedies for healing wounds, burns and ulcers. Taken internally as a tea it has a soothing, healing action on the lining of the digestive tract. A double-strength tea used externally helps to reduce problems from fungal infections of the skin and will heal minor wounds, burns and ulcers. It is worth using regularly on varicose veins – although it cannot be guaranteed to return them to normal, it will help to reduce the aching and discomfort that they cause and prevent further deterioration. It has a very soothing effect on haemorrhoids as well. It is worth trying in any case of skin irritation and inflammation too. The ointment is just as effective as the lotion, and is one of the most popular and easily available herbal preparations.

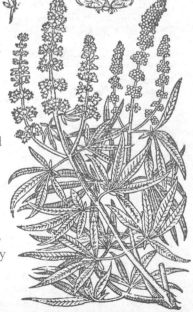

Combines well with: witch-hazel as an application to varicose veins, and with witch-hazel and lesser celandine for haemorrhoids. For skin rashes and irritation mix marigold and chickweed ointments. For digestive problems try it with meadowsweet and marshmallow for an excellent healing combination. Mix it with St John's wort for a general skin/healing combination.

Culpeper says: *'They strengthen the heart exceedingly, are very expulsive, and little less effectual in the small pox and measles than saffron. The flowers, either green or dried, are much used in possets, broths and drinks, being comfortable to the heart and spirits and expelling any malignent or pestilential quality which might annoy them.'*

MARSHMALLOW

Althaea officinalis

Family: malvaceae. **Part used:** root and leaf. **Constituents:** mucilage. **Action:** demulcent, diuretic, expectorant (root). **Helps to:** soothe inflammation in stomach and lungs, reduce digestive disturbances and discomfort, calm skin irritation (external application).

Historical notes: In the Middle East, the marshmallow is known as an emergency source of food, especially in times of famine. The root is said to be quite palatable, fried with onions and butter. The tender tops of the plant are still eaten in France as an addition to green salads. Most people will be familiar with the marshmallow as a soft and sticky sweet which was indeed once made from the root of the plant; this has now been replaced by cheaper, alternative materials.

Present uses: I prefer using the root to the leaf as there is far more of the mucilage here. In fact there is so much that the preparation I make has only half the usual amount of root in it, otherwise the results are too gooey to use! It is excellent in any mixture given to help the digestion: the mucilage mimics the action of the mucus produced naturally by the stomach and puts a soothing, protective surface over the irritated membrane. This calms the inflammation and enables the healing processes to work more efficiently.

There is a reflex calming action on the lungs via the stomach. Thus marshmallow helps as a soothing expectorant, reducing inflammation and loosening phlegm. Used externally the benefits are similar: there is a calming and protective action on any skin inflammation.

Combines well with: *liquorice, marigold and meadowsweet for stomach problems, especially in connection with overacidity and ulcers. Mix it with *elecampane, white horehound or *coltsfoot to help soothe an irritating cough. Combine it with slippery elm powder or fenugreek for applying to skin inflammation.

Culpeper says: *'The roots are of special use for coughs, hoarseness, shortness of breath, and wheezings, being boiled in honeyed water or wine, and drunk, and with good success used by them that have excoriations in the guts, or the bloody flux, by moderating the violence of sharp fretting humours, easing the pains and healing the soreness'.*

C A U T I O N

Do not take liquorice or elecampane in pregnancy.
Long-term use of coltsfoot is not advised.

MEADOWSWEET *Filipendula ulmaria*

Family: rosaceae. **Part used:** leaves. **Constituents:** salicylate compounds. **Action:** soothing to the stomach, mild urinary antiseptic, antirheumatic, astringent. **Helps to:** calm digestive disturbance, reduce arthritic inflammation.

Historical notes: Before carpets were invented, fragrant plants were scattered over the bare floor and meadowsweet was one of the favourites. With its strongly aromatic but sweet smell it must have brightened many a dark medieval homestead.

Present uses: Meadowsweet tea is one of the most reliable remedies for helping digestive problems. It contains valuable minerals that neutralize excess stomach acids, and is therefore the main treatment for problems like indigestion, heartburn and ulcers. It is also worth trying for nausea and diarrhoea, particularly in children where a gentle but effective treatment is required. Its other constituents include a useful amount of salicylates, which are the natural equivalent of aspirin. Purified aspirin can be very harsh on the stomachs of many people, but the overall combination of constituents in meadowsweet is so soothing that this problem never occurs when the whole plant is used. It is therefore suitable for its anti-inflammatory action for people with aspirin-sensitive stomachs who have problems with arthritis and rheumatism.

CAUTION

Do not take celery seeds or liquorice in pregnancy.

Combines well with: marigold and marshmallow for digestive problems; or with *liquorice, particularly to help an ulcer; or with agrimony if the upset involves diarrhoea. Mix with *celery seeds for arthritis and rheumatism.

Culpeper says: *'It is very effectual to open the urinary passages, and to help the stranguary, and all other pains of the bladder and reins, and to expel the stone and gravel, by taking the roots in powder and mixed with honey are good to be taken by those whose stomachs are swollen, breaking and expelling the wind which was the cause thereof.'*

MOTHERWORT *Leonurus cardiaca*

Family: labiatae. **Part used:** leaves. **Constituents:** alkaloids, bitters, volatile oil. **Action:** heart tonic, female reproductive system tonic. Helps to: support the normal functioning of the heart, reduce high blood pressure, normalize menstrual disturbances.

Historical notes: The name of the plant comes from two sources. The genus, *Leonurus*, is Greek for lion's tail, which refers to the appearance of the plant. While the species name *cardiaca* may suggest that the plant has some use as a treatment for heart disease, it is actually a corruption of the Latin *cordiaca*, referring to the fact that the leaves used to be made into a syrup or cordial.

Present uses: In all problems of heart function, motherwort tea will have a supportive action almost akin to a nutritional tonic. It doesn't either speed up or slow down the heart rate, but helps to make the overall function stronger and more efficient. It helps to bring down a high blood pressure, and recent research indicates that it could have the ability to improve the circulation in other ways.

The other valuable action is the normalizing influence it seems to have on a wide range of problems associated with the female reproductive system. Take it to help with premenstrual problems and irregular or painful periods. It can help in cases of endometriosis, and is recommended in the last month of pregnancy (but not before this time) to act as an aid to labour and birth.

Combines well with: hawthorn for problems of the circulation, and yarrow as well if the blood pressure is high. Mix it with black haw to help with painful periods, and with *red sage and St John's wort for menopausal hot flushes.

Culpeper says: *'The powder therefore to the quantity of a spoonful, drunk in cold wine, is a wonderful help to women in sore travail, as also for suffocation or risings of the mother; and from these effects it most likely got the name of mother-wort. It also provoketh urine, and women's courses; cleanseth the chest of cold phlegm oppressing it, and killeth worms in the belly.'*

C A U T I O N

Do not take red sage if you may be pregnant rather than starting the menopause.
Do not take motherwort in the first eight months of pregnancy.

MYRRH *Commiphora molmol*
Family: burseraceae. **Part used:** resin (dried gum). **Constituents:** resin, gum, volatile oil, bitters. **Action:** antimicrobial, astringent, carminative, expectorant, anticatarrhal, antiseptic. **Helps to:** support the body's fight against infections, heal minor wounds.
Historical notes: Myrrh has been prized for thousands of years for its healing and preserving properties as well as its use in perfumes and incense. The ancient Egyptians used it for embalming their pharaohs, and thought so highly of it that they credited it with the ability to bring the dead back

to life. It appears in the Bible in the holy oil of the Israelites and was one of the gifts brought by the Wise Men to the infant Jesus.

Present uses: It is the most useful of antiseptic remedies. It can be bought at most chemist shops as tincture of myrrh, which is still a standard pharmaceutical preparation. Use this neat on mouth ulcers – it will sting for a moment, but this soon goes and the ulcers will then heal much more quickly. It can also be applied neat to the gums as a treatment for infections and as an emergency temporary treatment for toothache. Alternatively, dilute the tincture: add half a teaspoon of it to a tablespoon of warm water and use it as a mouthwash. If you have a sore throat you can use it as a gargle. The same dilution can be used to clean minor cuts and grazes, where it will act as an antiseptic and also help promote healing processes in the skin. It can be taken internally to help against infections – it has the ability to stimulate the activity of the immune system. Take very small doses – about an eighth of a teaspoon well diluted in water – as the taste is very 'antiseptic'!

Combines well with: comfrey ointment applied to a wound after it has been bathed with tincture of myrrh, to maximize the rate of healing.

Culpeper says: *'Being mixed with wine and nettles it is very efficacious in most of the diseases peculiarly incident to the female sex.'*

NETTLES (STINGING)
Urtica dioica
Family: urticaceae. **Part used:** leaves. **Constituents:** flavonoids, silicic acid. **Action:** diuretic, haemostatic. **Helps to:** eliminate waste products via the kidneys, improve the condition of the skin, reduce arthritis and rheumatic problems.

Historical notes: The humble nettle, usually thought of only as an unpleasant, stinging weed, has served people well in many guises for hundreds of years. The fibres of the mature nettle are equal to those of flax and produce an excellent linen-type cloth. This was used in Britain well into the eighteenth century; on the continent, especially Germany, nettles were used to manufacture cloth for uniforms in the First World War. The value of nettles as a food has also been well known and many references to this appear in literature; for instance, in 1661 Samuel Pepys wrote that he enjoyed a 'serving of nettle porridge'. Nettle beer was brewed in Britain for hundreds of years until replaced by hops in the fifteenth century.

Nettle fritters are a traditional way of eating nettles; they are tasty and nourishing and very easy to make. Here is a modern version of the recipe, which makes eight good-sized fritters:

225g (8 oz) young nettle tops ~ 1 medium onion
vegetable oil ~ 115g (4 oz) porridge oats
60g (2 oz) grated cheese ~ 1 tbsp soy sauce
salt and pepper

Wash the nettle tops (be careful - they may retain their sting at this stage). Chop the onion very finely and sauté gently in a little oil for a few minutes before adding the nettles and half a cup of water. Continue to cook slowly, stirring now and then until the nettles are soft and much reduced. Continue cooking for a few minutes, then remove from the heat and stir in the oats and the grated cheese. Add the soy sauce and salt and pepper to taste. Leave for a minute or two, then pat into fritter shapes and fry gently on both sides for a few minutes until golden brown. Served with a mixed salad, these fritters make a delicious and nutritious meal.

Present uses: Nettles have always been valued for their nutritional as much as their medicinal benefits. In some parts of Britain it is traditional to cook the young tops as a vegetable in spring, preparing them in a similar way to spinach. Their high mineral content makes them extremely nutritious and the taste is very palatable. Alternatively they can be made into a tea and taken as part of a 'spring tonic', helping the organs of elimination to remove waste products that may build up over the winter periods of inactivity. This is especially helpful for skin problems such as eczema and irritating rashes. Dried nettles should be used from midsummer onwards for this purpose, as most of the benefit from the fresh plant is lost after it has flowered.

The herb is also useful for arthritis and rheumatism. It helps the kidneys get rid of the acids that can aggravate these problems, thus reducing the causes of the inflammation. It has proved to be very helpful for gout, which is specifically due to the accumulation of uric acid at the inflamed joints.

Combines well with: oregon grape and clivers to help skin problems. Mix nettles with *celery seeds to help arthritis and rheumatism.

CAUTION

Do not take celery seeds in pregnancy.

Culpeper says: *'Nettle tops, eaten in spring, consume the phlegmatic superfluities in the body which the coldness and moisture of winter hath left behind. The decoction also, or the seed also provoketh urine, and has hardley ever been known to fail for expelling the gravel and stone from the reins and the bladder. The juice of the leaves or the decoction from them, or of the roots, is very good to wash either old, rotten or stinking sores, fistulas and gangrenes, scabs, manginess and itch in any part of the body.'*

OREGON GRAPE *Mahonia aquifolium*

Family: berberidaceae. **Part used:** root. **Constituents:** alkaloids. **Action:** anticatarrhal, anti-emetic (reduces tendency to vomiting), mild cholagogue and laxative. **Helps to:** improve liver function.

Historical notes: This shrub was introduced into the UK from America in the early nineteenth century. It is a relative of the popular *Berberis* genus found in so many gardens and several varieties, notably 'Charity', are grown as winter-flowering shrubs.

Present uses: Its main property is its ability to stimulate liver function. Taken as a decoction, this will help the digestion. It is a useful remedy in the treatment of all digestive disturbances where nausea and lack of appetite are involved. It is also valuable indirectly, through its liver actions, in helping skin problems and some types of headache. The liver is a most important detoxifying organ; as such, if it can be stimulated to more efficient activity, often apparently unrelated diseases can be successfully treated. Thus oregon grape is worth taking in cases of eczema and psoriasis, and even for unexplained skin rashes. With a migraine, it is often helpful to take a liver-stimulating remedy. Oregon grape is ideal, as it is effective but gentle.

Combines well with: nettles, red clover and clivers to help skin problems.

PASSION FLOWER *Passiflora incarnata*

Family: passifloraceae. **Part used:** leaves. **Constituents:** alkaloids and flavonoids. **Action:** relaxing, antispasmodic, anodyne. **Helps to:** reduce anxiety, nervous and muscular tension, ease aches and pains.

Historical notes: Despite its name, the passion flower does not, unfortunately, have any romantic connections. It is named for its appearance, which is reminiscent of the passion of Christ: the stamens form the crown of thorns and the distinctive three-branched stigma in the centre resembles the three nails. It was introduced to Britain from the West Indies and South America in the late seventeenth century.

Present uses: This is one of my most-used remedies, as it has a very reliable calming and relaxing effect. Take it as a tea to help calm anxiety and nervous tension. To help relieve insomnia, take one cup in the middle of the evening and a second one just as you go to bed. It can help reduce the physical discomfort that often accompanies feelings of anxiety, such as palpitations, trembling and sweating. I have also found it to be one of the most effective remedies for reducing pain in problems like neuralgia, shingles and headaches.

Combines well with: scullcap for the general calming and relaxing properties of both remedies. For insomnia passion flower is often combined with valerian; these two remedies are available together in tablet form. For its pain-relieving action, mix it with St John's wort.

CAUTION

Do not take passion flower during pregnancy.

PEPPERMINT *Mentha piperita*
Family: labiatae. **Part used:** leaves. **Constituents:** volatile oil, flavonoids. **Action:** antispasmodic, carminative, diaphoretic, local anaesthetic. **Helps to:** improve the digestion, reduce flatulence and colic, reduce a high temperature, ease muscular cramps.

Historical notes: A Mediterranean plant, peppermint has been used for thousands of years and many references to it can be found in the classical literature of ancient Greece and Rome. It is named after a nymph of Roman mythology, Minthe. Pluto, the god of the underworld, fell in love with her, so his jealous wife Proserpine turned her into the plant which now bears her name.

Sprays of mint adorned dinner tables in ancient times, its clean and fresh smell welcoming hungry guests. It was also used extensively in cooking to flavour both food and wine, and is still taken as a tea in many Mediterranean and Eastern countries. In the UK it has been cultivated since the eighteenth century, and was mainly grown in the home counties - you may remember the famous 'Mitcham mint' confectionery - and Lincolnshire. Although some of the crop was dried, most went to make oil of peppermint. This has a range of uses in cookery, medicine and perfumery.

Present uses: Peppermint tea is one of the best known of all herbal remedies. It is a popular summertime drink, when many people find the cooling effect of the constituent menthol is preferable to the taste of ordinary tea. It is an outstanding remedy for digestive problems. Many people who know little about herbal medicine still know that sucking a mint sweet helps with indigestion. Taking the tea is far more beneficial. It reduces flatulence, indigestion and colic, and helps nausea and liver problems. It is also worth taking at the onset of a feverish cold, as its diaphoretic properties help reduce a high temperature. Catarrhal problems may be reduced by taking peppermint both as a tea and as a *steam inhalation. Pure menthol crystals can be bought for this purpose, and they certainly have a clearing effect on the nasal passages, but I think they have a rather harsh action: it is better to use one or two drops of oil of peppermint in water, or simply to inhale the vapours of a double-strength tea. Another action is the antispasmodic effect on muscles: oil of peppermint is an old remedy for cramps. Used externally it helps to reduce the pain of headaches and neuralgia.

Combines well with: chamomile or caraway to help the digestion. For colds and catarrh, mix it with elderflowers. For external use on tired, aching muscles combine it in a lotion with lavender and rosemary. This also makes a pleasant application to the temples to relieve headaches.

Culpeper says: *'It helpeth a cold liver; strengtheneth the belly and stomach: causeth digestion; stayeth vomiting and the hiccough; is good against the gnawing of the heart; provoketh apetite; taketh away obstructions of the liver, and stirreth up bodily lust.'*

CAUTION

Some people with asthma may find that steam is irritating to their chests. Steam inhalations should not be used in these cases.

PSYLLIUM SEEDS *Plantago psyllium*
Family: plantaginaceae. **Part used:** seeds or husks. **Constituents:** mucilage. **Action:** demulcent, laxative. **Helps to:** soften and lubricate the stools, making bowel-motions easier and more regular, thus relieving both diarrhoea and constipation; calms irritable bowel syndrome; reduces blood cholesterol levels.

Historical notes: The plant is native to the countries bordering the Mediterranean; the closely related ispaghula seed originates from India and Pakistan. It has always been used in these countries for helping to ease bowel problems.

Present uses: It seems too good to be true that there is a remedy that helps relieve both diarrhoea and constipation, but psyllium does achieve this. It works simply because of the consistency of the gel that forms when the seeds or husks are added to water. When you prepare it, add about a teaspoon or so of psyllium to a tumbler of water. Leave it for half an hour and the gel will form, but it will still be quite fluid with this amount of water. Drink it, and repeat the dose up to three times a day if required (though once or twice a day at the most is probably all that you will need to relieve constipation – more may be needed if you have very loose motions). The seeds have no taste, so they are not unpleasant to take, but if you prefer to add them to diluted juice rather than plain water by all means do so.

When the gel enters the digestive tract it mixes with the food passing through and helps to give it a soft but well-formed consistency: either a very hard stool or an excessively loose stool is thus avoided. This makes psyllium an ideal treatment for problems like irritable bowel where the functioning of the bowel can swing from one extreme to the other. A further benefit of the gel is that it soaks up bile in the digestive tract. This leads to the formation and ejection of more bile, which requires the breakdown of cholesterol. Thus taking psyllium regularly helps clear cholesterol from the body.

Combines well with: slippery elm (taken separately, as it is prepared differently) in cases of diarrhoea. To lower cholesterol levels more effectively, take dandelion root and ginger as well as psyllium.

RASPBERRY LEAVES *Rubus ideaeus*

Family: rosaceae. **Part used:** leaves, fruit. **Constituents:** tannins (leaves), Vitamin C (fruit). **Action:** astringent, uterine tonic. **Helps to:** soothe an inflamed throat, calm diarrhoea, help period pains, help the function of the uterus during birth.

Historical notes: The name is Latin for 'the bramble that grows on Mount Ida'. The plant grows wild throughout Europe. The fruits have been used for their Vitamin C content and have long been known as a treatment for scurvy. Raspberry vinegar was taken as a delicious drink, particularly for colds and sore throats. It can be made as follows. Add 1.1 litres (2 pints) of wine vinegar to 450g (1lb) of fresh raspberries in a crock (don't use metal vessels). Soak overnight, then strain off the liquid and add it to another 450g (1lb) of raspberries. Soak this overnight, and repeat the following day with yet another 450g (1lb) of raspberries. When this has soaked overnight the preparation has reached the correct strength. Then add 450g (1lb) of sugar to every 570ml (1 pint) of liquid, heat the mixture gently to dissolve it, skim the surface, allow to cool and then bottle it. Dilute it as you would fruit squash before drinking.

Present uses: Its astringent properties make raspberry leaf tea useful to soothe inflammation in the throat and digestion. As you swallow the tea, it reduces discomfort and swelling in the throat, so sip it slowly for the best results. It is reputed to be most effective against diarrhoea if taken cold.

Raspberry has a great reputation for helping with menstrual problems and is well worth taking by women who have irregular, heavy or painful periods, or premenstrual problems as well. The use of raspberry leaf tea in the later stages of pregnancy was well-known folklore until recently. It seems to help the uterus work efficiently with minimum pain. It should not be taken until the last month of pregnancy, because any stimulating action on the uterus could be dangerous before that time.

Combines well with: *red sage for a gargle in cases of tonsillitis or sore throats. Use it with agrimony to reduce diarrhoea.

C A U T I O N

*Do not take raspberry leaves in the first eight months of pregnancy.
Do not take red sage at all in pregnancy.*

R E D   C L O V E R   *Trifolium   pratense*
Family: leguminosae. **Part used:** flowers. **Constituents:** glycosides, flavonoids, volatile oil. **Action:** alterative, expectorant. **Helps to:** calm inflammatory skin disease, ease coughs.

Historical notes: This plant is a common weed in lawns and is found abundantly in the UK. Children have always liked to pick the flower heads and suck the base of each separate floret to get the drop of sweet nectar found there.

Present uses: This is one of the most useful herbs to take as a tea for skin problems like eczema and psoriasis. Its mode of action is mysterious, as one of the remedies known traditionally as an alterative, but it is completely safe and usually very effective. Try it for rashes of non-specific origin too. It is also helpful for coughs and chest infections, helping to loosen tight phlegm and ease discomfort.

Combines well with: clivers and nettles and oregon grape for skin problems, and with white horehound or ★elecampane for coughs.

Culpeper says: *'The juice dropped into the eyes is a familiar medicine with many country people to take away the pin and web (as they call it) in the eyes; it also allayeth the heat and blood shooting of them.'*

C A U T I O N

Do not take elecampane in pregnancy.

RED SAGE *Salvia officinalis*

Family: labiatae. **Part used:** leaves. **Constituents:** volatile oil, tannin, resin. **Action:** astringent, antiseptic, carminative. **Helps to:** soothe a sore throat, fight off throat infections.

Historical notes: The sages are native to the Mediterranean countries, but have been known in the UK at least since the sixteenth century. They seem quite hardy enough to survive in the British climate and do best when growing in a sunny position. The green (sometimes known as white or garden) sage is the species most often seen growing in gardens and is used as the culinary herb, but the species used medicinally is the red sage. This makes a most attractive garden plant itself. The botanical name comes from the Latin word *salvere*, meaning to save, which indicates how highly its therapeutic properties were valued. An old saying is 'He that would live for aye,/Must eat Sage in May'. It had a reputation for helping to sharpen the wits and treat nervous problems, and to treat 'the bitings of serpents'.

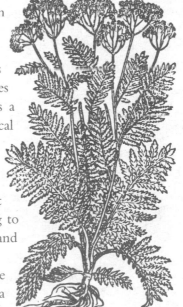

Present uses: Red sage tea is the prime astringent remedy used for its local actions on a sore throat. It has a very pungent taste, so make the tea fairly dilute to start with and increase the strength later if you wish. It helps to reduce swelling and discomfort, and the oil in the plant has an antiseptic effect, helping to fight the infection. Sip it slowly to get the maximum benefit, as the longer it is present in the throat the better the results. Alternatively, use it as a gargle and mouthwash: it can help with gum problems when taken regularly in this way. The tea is also a good digestive remedy, taken to reduce flatulence and colic. Its other main use is in several 'female' problems. It seems to help reduce excessive perspiration when taken internally, and is very effective for helping most women who have severe hot flushes as part of the menopause. It also helps to reduce the production of breast milk, so can be taken by lactating women at the stage when they want to reduce breast-feeding.

Combines well with: *raspberry leaves and *thyme to help sore and infected throats, and with *motherwort during the menopause.

CAUTION

Do not take red sage or thyme in pregnancy.
Do not take raspberry leaves in the first eight months of pregnancy.
Do not take motherwort if you may be pregnant rather than starting the menopause.

Culpeper says: *'The juice of sage taken in warm water, helpeth an hoarseness and cough. Gargles likewise are also made with sage, rosemary, honey-suckles and plantane, boiled in wine or water with some honey or alum put thereto, to wash sore mouths and throats.'*

ROSEMARY *Rosmarinus officinalis*

Family: labiatae. **Part used:** leaves and stems. **Constituents:** volatile oil, resin, bitters. **Action:** carminative, antispasmodic, nervine, antimicrobial.

Helps to: improve the digestion, relax tension, ease depression, fight infections.

Historical notes: Rosemary was once used as a symbol of lasting love between sweethearts, probably due to its reputation as a tonic for improving the memory. At weddings it was used to deck the church and was often to be found woven into the bride's bouquet. After the wedding it took on a very different meaning; it was said that where rosemary flourished the wife was master of the house. I have a thriving specimen growing in my front garden.

It was used to treat digestive problems, gout and mental disorders. It was thought to preserve youthfulness if the scent was inhaled, and items made of rosemary wood were prized for this. It also had a reputation for curing baldness.

Present uses: Although rather pungent-tasting, a rosemary tea made to an acceptable strength is an excellent remedy for the digestion. It helps to calm flatulence and colic, promotes the appetite and stimulates liver function. It has a good reputation for helping with problems caused by stress, including anxiety and depression. Take it to alleviate headaches, and apply it externally over the temples as well.

Externally applied, rosemary helps local circulation and relaxes muscle tension. The oil is more often used in this way than the tea. It can be bought at most good herb/health shops. Add a few drops of the oil to a teaspoonful of almond oil when you use it, as it is too strong to use neat. (The problem is not that it has a harmful effect on the skin, but that once it is absorbed into the body it has to be broken down and eliminated. Using the neat oil introduces a comparatively large amount of this potent substance into the body and can either put a strain on the organs of elimination or cause the build-up of an excessive amount of it.) There seems to be some truth in its reputation for promoting hair growth, possibly due to the camphor content of the oil. Massage the diluted oil into the scalp regularly, or use the tea as a lotion. It can also be added to the final rinsing water when the hair is washed.

Combines well with: wood betony for headaches and anxiety/depression problems. For external use, mix it with lavender oil in a suitable diluting oil. To improve the condition of the scalp and help hair growth, combine it with nettles. Take the combined tea internally and add oil of rosemary to nettle tea as a lotion applied to the scalp.

Culpeper says: '*The decoction therof in wine helpeth the cold distilations of rheum in the eyes, and all other diseases of the head and brain, as the giddiness or swimming therein, drowsiness or dulness of the mind and senses, the dumb palsey, or loss of speech, the lethargy and falling sickness. To be both drunk and the temples bathed therein.*'

CAUTION

Do not take rosemary in pregnancy.

Sage see Red Sage

St John's Wort

Hypericum perforatum

Family: hypericaceae. **Part used:** leaves and flowers. **Constituents:** volatile oil, flavonoids, astringent substances. **Action:** nervine, astringent, promotes healing of skin. **Helps to:** calm nervous tension, heal minor wounds and burns, reduce menopause symptoms.

Historical notes: This plant grows as a weed throughout the UK and Europe. It had a reputation for being a magic plant and was believed to protect against evil spirits, as it was thought they could not bear being near it. It was always easy to identify among numerous other species of *Hypericum*, because if a leaf is held up to the light many perforations can be seen as dots which let the light through – hence the name *perforatum*.

Present uses: Internally a tea made of the leaves and flowers is a good remedy to calm nervous tension. It is used particularly for the emotional problems that some women experience at the menopause. Also, it seems to have a pain-reducing effect without having any of the disadvantages of orthodox painkillers. Try it for problems like neuralgia, sciatica and headaches. Recent research shows that tincture of St John's wort has significant anti-infection properties, making it useful against some viruses where there is little help from other medication. The active constituents are not extracted by water, though, so the tea does not have the same effect.

Externally the infused oil prepared from the leaves and flowers makes an excellent healing application for minor wounds and burns. Try it also on muscle strains, sprains and arthritic joints. Gently massage it onto the temples to relieve headaches, and apply it over areas of neuralgia.

Combines well with: wood betony or scullcap for nervous debility, or with *motherwort for menopause problems. Externally, alternate it with marigold to heal burns and with comfrey for muscle or joint problems.

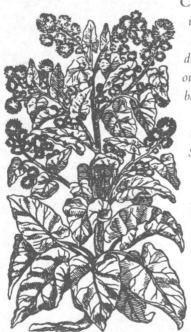

Culpeper says: *'It is by no means the least valuable for its efficacy in the cure of wounds, hurts or bruises by being boiled in wine and drunk, if the complaint is inwardly, or, if outwardly, by converting it into an oil, ointment, bath or lotion.'*

SCULLCAP

Scutellaria lateriflora

Family: labiatae. **Part used:** leaves and stem. **Constituents:** flavonoid, glycosides, bitters, tannins. **Action:** nervine, anodyne. **Helps to:** calm nervous tension and anxiety; reputed to help prevent epileptic seizures.

Historical notes: There are numerous species of scullcap. Two are found wild in the UK, though these are not used medicinally. One of the North American scullcaps, specifically the lateriflora, is the highly prized nervine remedy. It has been known in America as 'madweed', having been used in the past to treat rabies and convulsions.

Present uses: Scullcap is one of the remedies I use most frequently for a wide range of problems involving the nervous system. It helps with problems of physical and psychological origin. Take a tea to help against infections like shingles and other herpes viruses, and for inflammation of the nerves such as neuralgia or sciatica. It is worth trying as an additional treatment for epilepsy or convulsions. As a convalescent remedy it will help lift the depression and debility that some people suffer after 'flu or other fevers.

Take it also to help counteract the effects of stress: it aids the reduction of nervous tension, anxiety, headaches and insomnia.

Combines well with: *passion flower for a good general relaxing combination, or with vervain during convalescence and debility. Use it with cramp bark for muscle tension problems.

C A U T I O N

Do not take passion flower during pregnancy.

SENNA *Cassia acutifolia* or *angustifolia*
Family: leguminosae. **Part used:** leaves and fruits (known as 'pods').
Constituents: laxative anthraquinones.
Action: cathartic laxative. **Helps to:** stimulate bowel activity.

Historical notes: Senna is a native plant of Egypt and the Sudan and was used by Arab physicians before becoming known in Europe. It has been cultivated in Britain since the seventeenth century. It is still widely used as an over-the-counter laxative and prescribed by many medical practitioners for short-term use.

Present uses: Senna leaves can be made into a tea which, if taken at night, will stimulate a bowel-motion the following morning. If the pods are used, three to six of the Alexandrian variety, or double this number of the milder Tinnevelly variety, should be soaked in a cupful of warm water for eight hours and then taken at night. It takes this time for the remedies to work, as the active constituents are released as they pass through the intestine. Their mode of action is to irritate the lining of the intestine, which provokes greater activity in the bowel. For this reason senna can sometimes cause griping and colic; it is best taken with one of the carminative remedies such as ginger or fennel to prevent this. This treatment should not be used long term, as it is treating the symptoms rather than looking for the cause of the problem. Also, the bowel can become 'lazy' and dependent on the strong stimulus of a laxative to work at all if the remedy is used for too long a time.

C A U T I O N

Senna is best avoided during pregnancy and should only be taken under medical supervision.

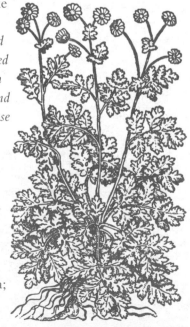

Combines well with: a carminative like ginger or fennel to avoid griping pains.

Culpeper says: *'It openeth obstructions and cleanseth and comforteth the stomach, being corrected with anise-seed, carraway-seed or ginger; it purgeth melancholy choler and phlegm, from the head and brain, lungs, heart, liver and spleen, cleansing those parts of evil humours.'*

SLIPPERY ELM
Ulmus fulva or rubra

Family: ulmaceae. **Part used:** powdered inner bark. **Constituents:** mucilage, starch and tannin. **Action:** demulcent, nourishing. **Helps to:** soothe an upset digestion, protect stomach and duodenal ulcers, calm diarrhoea; *externally*: calm inflamed skin.

Historical notes: This tree is indigenous to North America. The native Americans used to make a poultice from it to soothe damaged or inflamed skin and to 'draw' boils and abscesses. It was used by European settlers as a treatment for typhoid fever, to calm the severity of its digestive symptoms, during the epidemics of the eighteenth and nineteenth centuries, and also for severe chest infections like tuberculosis and pleurisy.

Present uses: There is nothing as soothing to an upset stomach as a drink made with slippery elm powder. It can be made with either water or milk, depending on your preference. Add one or two teaspoons of the powder to a little cold milk or water and stir until a smooth paste is formed. Top up with warm milk, stirring briskly, add a little sugar or honey and drink while it is still warm. It has a mild taste, and a texture slightly thicker than normal milky drinks, but is not at all unpleasant. Vary the consistency to suit your own taste. Alternatively, add it to a little plain yogurt and honey, stir to form a smooth consistency and eat this combination. You can buy capsules containing slippery elm too, and this is the most convenient way of getting the benefit if you can't make the drink. It takes a little longer to work, as the mucilage will be formed after the capsules have entered the stomach, but the end results will be the same.

The astringent properties of slippery elm help to calm inflammation, but most of the benefit is due to the mucilage that is formed when the powder comes into contact with a liquid. This gives a soothing, protective lining to the digestive tract as it passes through, thus calming inflammation. It reduces the tendency to diarrhoea before it reaches the bowel: anything that has a calming effect on the stomach works by reflexes in the gut to reduce overactivity further down.

Add slippery elm to poultices to get the right consistency so that they stay in place on the skin. It is soothing to inflamed skin in its own right, and can be a useful carrier for other less mucilaginous remedies.

Combines well with: chamomile and meadowsweet (taken as a separate drink, as they are prepared differently), to augment the soothing action of slippery elm. Psyllium seeds too (again taken separately) used with slippery elm will help to ease constipation.

Culpeper says: *'The decoction of the bark of the root mollifieth hard tumours, and the shrinking of the sinews being fomented therewith. The bark ground with brine or pickle until it cometh to the thickness of a poultice, and laid on the place pained with the gout, giveth great ease; and the decoction of the bark in water is exceeding good to bath such places as have been burned with fire.'*

THYME *Thymus vulgaris*

Family: labiatae. **Part used:** leaves and flowers. **Constituents:** volatile oil, bitters, tannins, resin. **Action:** antiseptic, antifungal, carminative, expectorant, antispasmodic. **Helps to:** fight infections, ease coughs and loosen tight phlegm, settle the digestion, calm flatulence and colic.

Historical notes: Common thyme originates from the wild thyme that is a native of the countries around the Mediterranean. It was established in the UK by the sixteenth century and survives well in the climate. Numerous varieties have been bred for the garden, with different appearances and scents, but the common thyme is the one specified for medicinal use. The name comes from the Greek word meaning 'to fumigate', so it has obviously been prized for its antiseptic properties for thousands of years. In the Middle Ages it was thought to impart courage to whoever drank a preparation of it. It has been used as a culinary herb since Greek and Roman times and as a favourite plant for bees, as it gives a characteristic fragrance to honey if planted near hives. It was used for all types of chest problems, including whooping cough. Most of the European crop is used to produce oil of thyme, which is used in the perfumery industry.

Present uses: Thyme tea is most used for its action against respiratory infections. It is worth taking in cases of sore throats, chest infections, tight coughs, etc. It helps to fight off the infection and to ease coughs and wheezing by loosening tight phlegm. A double-strength tea can be used as a gargle for sore throats and tonsillitis. At normal strength, taken internally, it is very effective in helping the digestion and has a reputation for promoting the secretions of the digestive system. It helps to reduce flatulence and colic.

Thyme has proved useful in helping to clear thrush in the mouth - use a double-strength tea as a gargle for this and then finally dilute and swallow a little. Laboratory research has shown that oil of thyme kills the candida organism.

Combines well with: *red sage or *raspberry leaves for a sore throat and with white horehound or *elecampane for coughs and chest infections. Combine the oil with diluted tincture of myrrh in a lotion to use against vaginal thrush.

CAUTION

Do not take thyme, red sage or elecampane in pregnancy.
Do not take raspberry leaves in the first eight months of pregnancy.

Culpeper says: *'This herb is a notable strengthener of the lungs; there is scarcely a better remedy growing for that disease in children which they commonly call the chin-cough. It purgeth the body of phlegm and is an excellent remedy for shortness of breath.'*

VALERIAN *Valeriana officinalis*
Family: valerianaceae. **Part used:** root. **Constituents:** volatile oil, alkaloids. **Action:** relaxant, antispasmodic. **Helps to:** calm nervous tension and

anxiety, promote normal sleep, reduce high blood pressure.

Historical notes: Valerian is a native plant of the UK. It has been used medicinally since the Middle Ages and is referred to in Anglo-Saxon writings. It is thought to be the plant known to the Greeks as fu (this is what you say when you smell the pungent root). It has always been highly prized for its relaxing properties. Cats love it: its smell makes them behave as if they were kittens again. Make a sachet containing valerian for your cat and it will play and roll about having great fun.

Present uses: A tea made of half to one teaspoonful of valerian root to one cupful of boiling water can be taken three times a day for problems of nervous tension, anxiety and/or *high blood pressure, particularly if this is caused by stress problems. If you take valerian tea to relieve insomnia, drink one cup in the middle of the evening and a second one about an hour before you want to get to sleep. It is also available in tablet form, which you may find more convenient. It has an excellent calming action and is worth trying for problems like neuralgia, muscle tension and panic attacks.

Combines well with: *passion flower for its general relaxing benefits. This is also a traditional combination to relieve insomnia and is available in tablet form from most herb/health shops.

Culpeper says: *'It is of special virtue against the plague, the decoction thereof being drunk, it helpeth also to expel the wind. The green herb, with the root taken fresh, being bruised and applied to the head, taketh away the pains and prickings therein and stayeth the rheums and thin distillations.'*

CAUTION

Seek professional help if you suspect a heart problem.
Do not take passion flower in pregnancy.

VERVAIN *Verbena officinalis*

Family: verbenaceae. **Part used:** leaves and stem. **Constituents:** bitters, tannins, volatile oil, glycosides. **Action:** nervine, antispasmodic. **Helps to:** calm nervous tension, lift depression, improve the digestion, aid recovery after debilitating illness.

Historical notes: This plant was used in religious rituals in pre-Christian days – the Druids considered it to have a purifying influence on its surroundings. Its alternative names include *herba sacra* and *herba Veneris* (herb of Venus – it had a reputation as an aphrodisiac, though I have not noticed this as a pronounced action on people taking the herb). The Romans held feasts called 'Verbenalia' in honour of the plant. Christian legend says it was vervain that staunched the wounds of Jesus during the Crucifixion and as such the plant deserved special respect. It had several medical uses, being taken for feverish infections; eye problems; to promote milk flow in lactating women; and to help to relieve urinary problems, particularly those involving kidney and bladder stones.

Present uses: Vervain is a valuable bitter and nervine remedy. It helps to promote the appetite and efficiency of the digestion and particularly the liver function. It has an almost nutritional restorative effect on the nervous system. This means that vervain tea is applicable to problems ranging from nervous tension and anxiety, to long-term stress resulting in nervous exhaustion, neuralgia, sciatica and shingles. Both actions are combined in its main use, which is as a restorative tonic in convalescence. Take it after a debilitating illness such as 'flu and digestive disturbances if a lot of weight has been lost and stamina needs restoring.

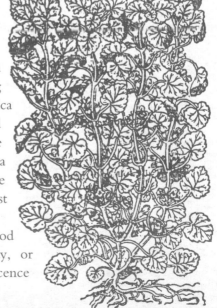

Combines well with: scullcap or wood betony for nervous tension or debility, or with white horehound for convalescence after a chest infection; and with an aromatic digestive remedy like caraway or cardamom to help the digestion.

Culpeper says: *'It consolidateth and healeth also all wounds both inward and outward and stayeth bleedings; and, used with some honey, healeth all old ulcers and fistulas in the legs or other parts of the body, as also those ulcers that happen in the mouth; or, used with old hog's grease, it helpeth the swellings and pains of the secret parts of man and woman, as also the piles and haemorrhoids.'*

WHITE HOREHOUND
Marrubium vulgare

Family: labiatae. **Part used:** leaf, stem and flowers. **Constituents:** bitters, alkaloids, flavonoids, volatile oil. **Action:** expectorant, bitter tonic. **Helps to:** stimulate the digestion, soothe a tight cough, ease phlegm production.

Historical notes: The name may come from the Hebrew word *marrob*, meaning a bitter juice. The plant is probably one of the bitter herbs taken by Jews at the Passover feast. It was thought to protect against magic charms and to help against bites by snakes and mad dogs. It has been used since Elizabethan times for its benefit against coughs and for its bitter tonic properties. Horehound candy was made by boiling the leaves to extract the juice, then adding enough sugar to the strained liquid to enable it to solidify when it cooled.

Present uses: This is one of my favourite remedies for coughs: it helps to loosen tight phlegm and has an excellent soothing effect on the membranes lining the lungs. Most people taking it as a tea find that their coughs and chest discomfort diminish steadily until they are well again. The bitter properties make it useful for chest infections where the appetite has been lost and I think of it as a useful convalescent remedy for people recovering from problems like bronchitis.

Combines well with: *elecampane, boneset, *thyme and *coltsfoot for chest problems. Add *gentian or vervain for a convalescent mixture to help people recovering from 'flu or chest infections.

C A U T I O N

Do not take elecampane or thyme in pregnancy.
Long-term use of coltsfoot is not advised.
Gentian should not be taken by people who have gastric or duodenal ulcers.

Culpeper says: *'The juice of the green herb being taken with honey, is a certain remedy for those that are pursey, or short winded, or have a cough, or are fallen into a consumption, either through long sickness or thin distillations of rheum upon the lungs. It helpeth to expectorate tough phlegm from the chest'*

WHITE WILLOW *Salix alba*

Family: salicaceae. **Part used:** bark. **Constituents:** salicylates, flavonoids, tannins. **Action:** anti inflammatory, astringent, reduces fever, painkiller. **Helps to:** reduce pain and inflammation in arthritis and rheumatism, bring down a high temperature. **Historical notes:** This species of willow is a native of central and southern Europe. The bark of young branches of various willows was used as a source of the anti-inflammatory salicylate compounds (generally known as 'aspirin') long before these substances were discovered, purified and artificially manufactured. **Present uses:** Use half to one teaspoonful of white willow bark to a cupful of boiling water to make willow tea. It is usually taken to relieve arthritis and rheumatism symptoms. It helps reduce both

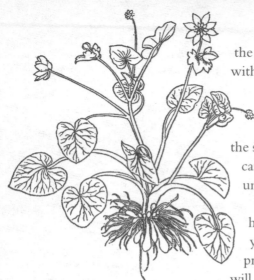

the pain and inflammation connected with these problems. Take it also to reduce period pains. Unlike pure aspirin, the salicylates as they are found in willow bark do not have the side-effects of stomach irritation and so can be tolerated by people who are unable to take pure aspirin.

The other benefit is the reduction of high temperatures: if remedies like yarrow and boneset don't solve the problem, willow bark almost certainly will. It can also be used as a general painkiller, to relieve occasional headaches, minor toothaches, etc.

Combines well with: *celery seeds to help relieve arthritis and rheumatism; and with St John's wort for its painkilling properties, in cases of headaches, neuralgia, etc.

C A U T I O N

Do not take celery seeds in pregnancy.

Culpeper says: *'The leaves being bruised and boiled in wine and drunk, stayeth the heat of lust. The decoction of the leaves or bark in wine takes away scurf, or dandruff, by washing the place with it.'*

WILD LETTUCE *Lactuca virosa*
Family: compositae. **Part used:** leaves. **Constituents:** bitters, alkaloids.
Action: relaxant. **Helps to:** calm nervous tension, promote sleep.
Historical notes: The name *Lactuca* comes from the Latin name for milk, because the sap of the plant is an opaque white colour. It grows wild throughout Europe. It has been used since the time of the Romans and was highly thought of as a restorative remedy. The dried sap, known as

'lactucarium', was collected for medicinal use in the past. It has always had a reputation for its relaxing effects, which extended to cultivated lettuces too: an old folk cure for insomnia was to simmer two lettuces in a pan of water and drink the resulting liquid.

Present uses: I think of wild lettuce as one of the stronger relaxing remedies and generally keep it for problems of insomnia and intractable pain. For conditions such as painful arthritis or period pains, or for an emergency treatment for earache, toothache, etc., a tea made from half to one teaspoon of the herb to one cupful of water can be taken three times a day. For insomnia, take a slightly stronger tea, using about one teaspoon of the herb to a cupful of water, once in the middle of the evening and again just before going to bed.

Combines well with: ^passion flower or valerian for a general strong relaxing effect and to relieve insomnia.

C A U T I O N

Do not take passion flower in pregnancy.

Culpeper says: *'The juice of lettuce mixed or boiled with oil of roses and applied to the forehead and temples, procureth sleep and easeth the headache; being boiled and eaten it helpeth loosen the belly: it helpeth digestion, quencheth thirst, increases milk in nurses and easeth the griping pains that come in the stomach or bowels from choler.'*

WITCH-HAZEL *Hamamelis virginiana*
Family: hamamelidaceae. **Part used:** bark, twigs, leaves. **Constituents:** *bark*: tannins; *leaf*: tannins, volatile oil, bitters. **Action:** astringent, anti-inflammatory, haemostatic. **Helps to:** reduce inflammation and pain, staunch blood flow.
Historical notes: The witch-hazel tree is indigenous to North America

and was used by the native Americans as a poultice to heal injuries and abscesses, boils, etc. After its introduction to the UK it was found to be so useful that a number of recognized pharmaceutical preparations were made from it, using both leaves and bark. The crude leaves and bark, tincture, ointments and suppositories were all readily available. Nowadays distilled witch-hazel is the best-known preparation. This is a clear, colourless liquid with a characteristic fresh, woody scent. It contains the soluble extracts of witch-hazel twigs in a base of alcohol (about 15 per cent) and water. A very useful gel form is also now available.

Present uses: Witch-hazel has a hundred and one uses and is the most valuable first-aid remedy. It is an effective astringent and helps reduce inflammation – there is less pain and swelling at the site of an injury as a result. Keep a bottle available, particularly if you have children, as it is ideal for treating minor injuries. The 'magic water' soothes bumps, bruises and sprains, helps to stop blood flow from minor cuts and grazes and reduces the pain of insect bites and stings. It can be applied to minor burns and is an excellent treatment for sunburn: place a piece of lint or other suitable material over the affected area, pour the witch-hazel over it and keep the cloth moist by adding more witch-hazel as it dries out. Treat a bruise or sprain similarly.

As well as its use on injuries, witch-hazel's astringent action can be used to good effect on areas of lax tissue such as varicose veins and haemorrhoids. Apply it regularly twice a day – it can't be guaranteed to cure the problem but it will certainly reduce discomfort and, with other steps as appropriate, will help to prevent any further deterioration. Various proprietary ointments as well as liquid preparations are available for this. Distilled witch-hazel should not be taken internally, but a tea made from the leaf can be: use half a teaspoon of the herb to a cup of water, to reduce digestive discomfort associated with diarrhoea.

Combines well with: arnica ointment on bruises. Use marigold (as a tea, mixed with distilled witch-hazel and applied as a lotion) for varicose veins and haemorrhoids. Lesser celandine can be usefully added to this combination. Mix agrimony herb and witch-hazel leaves as a tea to relieve diarrhoea.

WOOD BETONY
Betonica officinalis

Family: labiatae. **Part used:** leaves and flowers. **Constituents:** alkaloids. **Action:** nervine, anodyne. **Helps to:** calm nervous tension and anxiety, ease headaches.

Historical notes: This plant is a native of the UK and has been prized throughout Europe for its therapeutic properties. It was used by the physicians to the Roman emperors and by the common people alike. Its popularity has been maintained through the centuries whilst herbal medicine has been used and it is still considered one of the most valuable of nervines. It used to have the reputation of being a protection against evil spirits, devils, despair and 'fearful visions' - which may have originated in its use as a remedy to relieve states of depression. In previous times it was used as a wound-healing herb, as was the closely-related species known as the woundworts. Wounded animals were thought to understand its efficacy and to search it out to heal themselves.

Present uses: Of all the nervine remedies, wood betony is the one I use the most. It has a gentle supportive action and I know of no one who has found it doesn't suit them. It well deserves its historical reputation. Take a tea made of the leaves for any problem associated with the nervous system, whether of physical or psychological origin. For herpes infections such as shingles, it can reduce the discomfort and help the nerves back to a condition of normality. It is also helpful against inflammations like sciatica and neuralgia. Take it for nervous tension and anxiety states, for panic attacks and insomnia, depression and debility, or headaches (it has the best reputation of any single remedy for use against headaches).

Combines well with: scullcap or vervain and damiana because of their combined nervine actions.

Culpeper says: *'It helpeth those that loathe or cannot digest their meat, those that hath weak stomachs ... it helpeth the jaundice, falling sickness, the palsy, convulsions, or shrinking of the sinews; the gout and those that are inclined to dropsies; and those that have continual pains in the head ... all sorts of coughs or colds, wheezing or shortness of breath ... the decoction thereof made in wine and taken, killeth worms in the belly, openeth obstructions both of the liver and spleen ... it helpeth also to break and expel the stone either in the bladder or kidneys ... easeth the toothache. The green herb bruised, or the juice applied to any inward hurt ... will quickly heal and close it up.'*

YARROW *Achillea millefolium*

Family: compositae. **Part used:** leaves and flowers. **Constituents:** volatile oil, flavonoids, alkaloids, tannins. **Action:** anti–inflammatory, antispasmodic, bitter, diaphoretic; staunches blood flow. **Helps to:** improve the appetite and digestion, reduce the severity of fevers, improve the circulation and reduce blood pressure.

Historical notes: Yarrow is a native of the UK and was a familiar plant in the past: it has a wide range of common names throughout the country. Its use as a wound herb is attested by the following names: nosebleed, bloodwort, staunchweed, sanguinary. The botanical name comes from the story that the Greek hero Achilles used it to treat his wounded soldiers and there are numerous other references to its use on the battlefield. It has been known as a medicinal plant in Britain since Saxon times and was used internally and externally, both the fresh juice and as a tea. It had a rather sinister reputation for being associated with the devil and was used in techniques of divination. In folklore rituals it was placed under the pillow at night; the appropriate charm being spoken, an unmarried person would then dream of her or his future spouse.

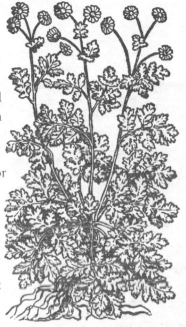

Present uses: A tea made of yarrow leaves has wide-ranging benefits. It is a good bitter tonic and helps settle the digestion and promote a feeling of general wellbeing. Take it at the first sign of the onset of a head-cold or 'flu and it will help the body's fight against these infections. It will reduce the severity of any fever symptoms, partly through its bitter action and partly by stimulating perspiration. It is also used for circulation problems, particularly *high blood pressure and varicose veins, as it may have a beneficial influence on the condition of the blood vessels. Externally the fresh juice or tea can be used as a directly applied lotion or as an additive to bathwater to soothe inflamed skin.

Combines well with: composition essence (see Chapter 9) or boneset, taken with yarrow every three hours, to help at the onset of head-colds or 'flu. It can be taken long term to help with circulation problems - it makes a good combination with hawthorn and *motherwort.

CAUTION

Seek professional help if you suspect a heart problem.
Do not take motherwort in the first eight months of pregnancy.

Culpeper says: *'An ointment of it cures wounds and is most fit for such as have inflammations. It stayeth the shedding of the hair, the head being bathed with the decoction of it. Inwardly taken, it helps the retentive faculty of the stomach and such as cannot hold their water. The leaves, chewed, ease the toothache.'*

YELLOW DOCK *Rumex crispus*

Family: polygonaceae. **Part used:** root. **Constituents:** anthraquinones, tannins. **Action:** alterative, mild laxative, liver tonic. **Helps to:** relieve constipation, improve liver function, calm inflammation of the skin.

Historical notes: There are several species of dock that grow wild in the UK. They all have similar constituents and broadly similar actions, but the one specified for medical use is the yellow, also known as curled, dock. It has always had a good reputation for relieving constipation without the griping effect that stronger laxatives can cause. It was used mainly as an alterative in the treatment of skin disease, but was occasionally used for acute problems; for example in cases of diphtheria.

The more familiar round-leaved dock had numerous uses as a folk remedy. Most people have tried putting the leaves on nettle stings. They were used as a covering for burns and blisters too, probably owing their efficacy to the tannins contained within the leaves. Country people also used the leaves for wrapping butter when it was to be transported to market.

In the north of England docks are the basis for a traditional pudding. The following recipe is still made in the Calder Valley and was passed on by Mrs Joan Laprell, who judges dock puddings in produce shows. It serves six.

Take a large supermarket carrier bag of young sweet docks (also known as red or water dock). Remove the stalks and chop the leaves. Boil two large chopped onions, add a handful of nettles (optional) and the docks and simmer for a fair time until most of the water has evaporated, leaving the mixture almost dry. Add two handfuls

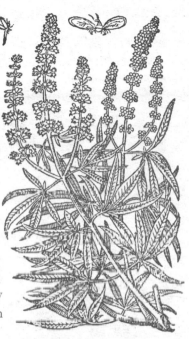

of medium oatmeal, stirring continuously, and salt and pepper as required. The pudding is traditionally eaten with bacon. It freezes well and is usually reheated by cooking in bacon fat. Some beaten egg is often mixed in with the pudding prior to reheating.

Present uses: Yellow dock is an excellent remedy for helping to improve liver and bowel function. Use it as a decoction in preference to *cascara or *senna when a gentle, less dramatic laxative action is required. Its main use is still in the treatment of skin disease, where its cleansing benefits often help reduce the overall severity of the inflammation very effectively, if indirectly. It is also useful in other conditions where a sluggish digestion may be having an adverse effect, such as arthritic and rheumatic disease.

Combines well with: burdock – mix two parts of yellow dock with one part of burdock root for an excellent decoction to take for skin problems like eczema and psoriasis. For constipation try taking psyllium seeds as well as yellow dock.

Culpeper says: '... *the yellow dock is best to be taken when either the blood or liver is afflicted by choler. The seed of most of the kinds [of docks], whether of the garden or field, doth stay fluxes of all sorts, the loathings of the stomach through choler and is helpful to those who spit blood. The root, boiled in vinegar, helpeth the itch, scabs and breaking out of the skin, if it be bathed therewith.*'

C A U T I O N

*Cascara and senna should not be taken in pregnancy.
Senna should only be taken under medical supervision.*

CHAPTER 7

COMMON AILMENTS: AN ALPHABETICAL GUIDE

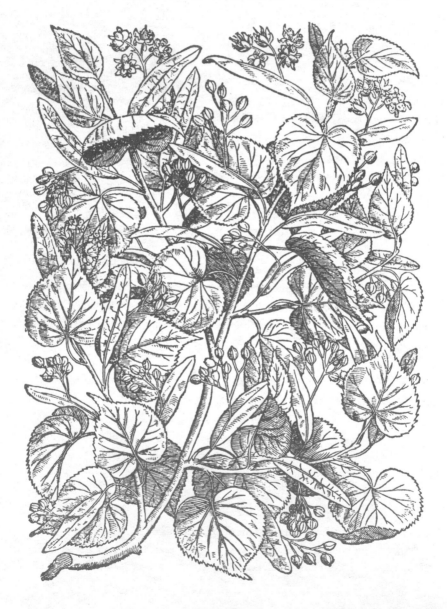

There are many common domestic ailments that can be treated very successfully with herbal remedies. Much of the information in this chapter would have been common knowledge a few generations ago. It has waned because of the immense increase in science and technology now applied to medicine, and because of most people's reliance on the National Health Service (an admirable social institution) rather than on the need for self-treatment. However, for the type of problem too minor for the need to consult a professional, there are plenty of effective herbal remedies to help. Let the guiding influence be whether or not you have an illness for which you would seek an over-the-counter pharmaceutical treatment: if this is the case, there is sure to be a herbal remedy that would be equally effective.

Although diet is not mentioned in every case, there are some illnesses where diet has been found to have a major effect on the outcome. Where specific foods are known to be helpful I have included them as part of the treatment. Where not, I think a good plain wholefood diet with a wide range of fruit and vegetables, moderate amounts of potatoes and cereal, and comparatively small amounts of dairy foods, meat and fish is what suits most people best. Not all foods suit all people, so this has to be adapted to the needs of each individual.

When it comes to problems that are beyond the scope of self-treatment and need professional attention, there are frequently herbal remedies that can contribute towards the recovery. All those mentioned in this chapter can be taken quite safely alongside orthodox treatment. There is also the option of having professional herbal treatment, which will give you access to a much wider range of remedies than you can obtain over the counter. Certain problems, even after successful treatment, may need to be monitored regularly by professionals to make sure that the improvement is maintained and no further problems are developing. Herbal remedies can be continued after orthodox treatment has been completed and are well-suited to long-term use. They can be thought of as a part of the diet that will help to improve your chances of staying healthy.

C A U T I O N

The information in this book is not intended to be an alternative to professional attention. If you are in any doubt about the nature of an illness, consult your doctor or a qualified herbal practitioner.

Chapter 5 explains how the remedies should be prepared: please read it before attempting to use any of them. Chapter 6 gives you more information about the individual remedies mentioned here: please read this too so that you know what their functions are and how they can help.

ABSCESSES

These very painful localized infections can have serious complications if they are not treated successfully, so I would always advise professional attention. Herbal treatment can help the body's natural way of fighting off the infection and can then help resolve the aftermath of the problem. The immune system stimulating remedies and the cleansing remedies that used to be referred to as 'blood purifiers' are very useful. They can help the body's attempts to defend itself against infection and rid itself of the products of the infection and inflammation. They stimulate the removal of waste products through the circulation, followed by their breakdown and elimination from the body. Echinacea is the prime anti-infective and cleansing remedy, with burdock and clivers also very valuable. Garlic can be taken internally and also applied to the site of the abscess. Follow a diet high in fresh fruit and vegetables to ensure an adequate supply of vitamins, minerals and fibre: these foods have always been thought of as natural cleansers.

CAUTION

Always seek professional help for an abscess.

ACNE

There are two components of this distressing problem. The underlying cause is usually an increase in the oil produced by the skin. In normal quantities this has a protective action, but when too much is produced it can encourage the bacteria (the second component) normally found on the skin to flourish and produce the painful red spots characteristic of acne. It is often connected with the hormone disturbances that occur during the teens, but can also be affected by stress and poor diet. Most orthodox treatment concentrates on getting rid of the bacteria with antibiotics. Herbal remedies that will also help with this are echinacea and garlic. There are numerous remedies that can help to reduce the oiliness of the skin and the resulting inflammation: try burdock, clivers and nettles as a tea. Witch-hazel can be used on the skin as an astringent: this will help to reduce oil production.

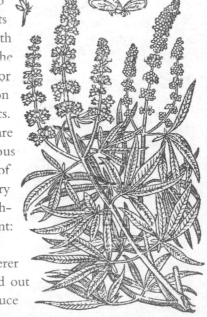

Certain foods may affect acne, and the sufferer may have to do some detective-work to find out what they are. My general advice is to reduce your intake of oily, fatty, sweet and refined or highly-processed foods, and increase that of fresh vegetables and fruits.

ALLERGIES

This covers a huge range of possible causes and reactions. Allergies are caused by the body's immune system reacting as if a harmful substance is attacking, against which it is mounting a defence. Possible triggers of this reaction include pollen and fungus spores that result in the nasal irritation, sneezing and asthma of hay fever; various foods that cause reactions in the digestive system, or skin problems like eczema; and chemicals such as detergents and oils that can produce contact dermatitis in the skin. Unless the allergic reaction is very straightforward it can be difficult to identify the cause: test diets may be necessary to check a range of possibilities. These diets require self-discipline and good organization to get useful results, and are probably best done under the guidance of a professional practitioner.

When the cause has been identified the best treatment is always to remove it as far as possible. This may be difficult if it is something in the environment, so trying to calm the body's reaction is the next line of treatment. Generally soothing anti-inflammatory remedies such as chamomile (used as a tea and also as a *steam inhalation for hay fever) and meadowsweet are useful.

C A U T I O N

Some people with asthma may find that steam is irritating to their chests. Steam inhalations should not be used in these cases.

Stress can aggravate an allergic reaction, so a gentle relaxing remedy like limeflowers may be helpful. Bitter tonics such as gentian may help to improve the digestive system's ability to cope with potentially allergenic substances.

ANXIETY

Considering the pressures of modern life, it is not surprising that anxiety is such a common problem. This feeling is an automatic part of the body's reactions to a threatening situation, caused by the production of the hormone called adrenaline. This is produced by the 'fight or flight' reactions of the nervous system and is designed to help get us out of a difficult situation quickly. Thousands of years ago it would have helped people to overcome or run away from danger such as a wild animal attacking, and even now it helps those like racing-drivers react quickly to dangerous situations. A slight feeling of anxiety is normal for people taking examinations or performing on stage, etc., and can even help them achieve better results by maximizing their alertness. It acts as an alarm that something is wrong and needs action to be put right. If it is the spur that gets you going to solve a problem, it has done its rightful job. The difficulty is that so many problems of daily life nowadays cannot be easily solved, so the anxiety can be a long-standing and very unpleasant experience. It can cause muscle tension, insomnia, tiredness, reduced ability to resist infections, digestive problems and many other disturbances of normal function.

Although herbal remedies can't make the problems go away, they can help to reduce the feeling of anxiety and also the severity of the symptoms it causes. The most gentle acting are chamomile and lemon balm (which are both particularly useful if there are problems with the digestion). Lavender is another good remedy, or if something stronger is required try *passion flower or valerian. The supply of the B group vitamins in the diet is very important, and can be obtained by taking a supplement of brewers' yeast tablets.

C A U T I O N

Passion flower should not be taken during pregnancy.

ARTHRITIS AND RHEUMATISM

This is a complex and variable condition, so there is only a limited amount of information that is likely to apply to all cases. It can be affected by a person's diet; citrus fruit, vinegar and pork products are common irritants. Some people with an allergy to wheat develop arthritis as a symptom. The circulation may be involved, as indicated by the problems becoming more severe in cold weather. Stress is often an influence too. All these factors need attention if the problem is to be dealt with successfully, so a consultation with a herbal practitioner may be required.

After these influences have been taken account of, the underlying approach is to cleanse the body of any irritants that may be adding to the inflammation. The classic remedy for this is *celery seeds (and celery stems should also be eaten as a vegetable as often as possible). These help the kidneys to work efficiently to eliminate waste products, and are almost specific for the accumulation of uric acid in the joints that characterizes gout. In addition, *feverfew seems to help in most cases. There are numerous supplements available that have helped different individuals. Eating oily fish such as salmon, sardines and mackerel regularly seems to have an anti-inflammatory effect, and the oil extracted from them, containing the active ingredient omega-3 fatty acids, is available as a supplement.

CAUTION

Celery seeds and feverfew should not be taken during pregnancy.
Be careful not to get cayenne in the eyes and keep away from broken skin.
Comfrey leaf and root can only be prescribed by a herbal practitioner.

There are several effective external treatments that can ease the symptoms, even if they don't cure the problem. Epsom salts in the bathwater has brought relief to many sufferers. An oil or lotion made from one part *cayenne to two parts each of cramp bark and *comfrey helps to improve the local circulation, relax muscle tension and promote healing. Naturopaths used to recommend a poultice made of kelp and/or cabbage leaves applied to the affected area once a day.

ASTHMA

This problem should *never* be treated just with home remedies – it is very variable in its severity, and an unexpected attack can be dangerous unless the right treatment is available quickly. It really does need professional assessment to establish a suitable treatment. I have included it in this book because there are several useful remedies that can act as auxiliary treatments, and in conjunction with professional treatment can help the condition of the airways. This can reduce the chances of the problem becoming severe.

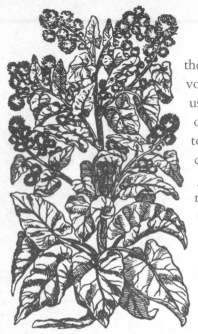

In asthma the rings of muscle that occur along the 'tubes' in the airways contract, reducing the volume of air that can pass through them. There is usually a distinct feeling of tightening in the chest of the sufferer, and sometimes a wheezing sound to breathing. Some people have a very characteristic dry cough as well, and a sticky, jelly-like phlegm may be produced. These reactions can be provoked in numerous situations, which have in common the result that the mucus membrane lining the airways becomes irritated. The cause may be a chest infection, or the breathing in of cold or polluted, smokey air. For hay fever sufferers, breathing in grass pollen can bring on an attack. The herbalist's approach is to use remedies that have a very soothing effect on the membranes of the lungs. First, any infection must be dealt with: garlic will be very helpful here. If cold weather is one of the factors involved, use a warming remedy like ginger or angelica as well. Then try regular doses of white horehound and *elecampane. These remedies calm irritation in the lungs and help produce a loose liquid phlegm that is easily coughed up. This will automatically help to relax the tightness in the chest and allow the lungs to work more efficiently.

C A U T I O N

Always seek medical attention for asthma.
Do not use elecampane in pregnancy.

ATHLETE'S FOOT

The feet are a perfect place for minor fungal infections to flourish, as they are usually covered by clothing and so are warm and moist. The herbal remedies that are most effective in clearing the infections are marigold, myrrh and thyme. These can be made into a footbath - use a strong infusion of marigold and thyme, and add about half a teaspoon of tincture of myrrh to this. Allow the preparation to cool to a temperature that feels pleasant, then soak the feet in it for about ten minutes. Do this once a day, or at least on alternate days. Distilled witch-hazel can be applied to the affected area to reduce itching and tenderness, and preparations made from the highly antifungal essential oil of the Australian tea tree (related to the eucalyptus, not to the Indian and Chinese tea bush used to make the everyday beverage) will also help to get rid of the infection. Generally, keep the feet clean and dry, and wear sandals to allow air to circulate round the feet whenever possible.

BILIOUS ATTACK

Although not technically accurate, this name is given to acute attacks of nausea, vomiting, digestive discomfort and the accompanying headache. It may be triggered by food sensitivities or overindulgence, as it is distinct from infections of the digestive system. The aim of treatment is to soothe the lining of the digestive tract and to calm the reactions of the inflamed stomach. Demulcent remedies such as marshmallow root and slippery elm powder are excellent for this - they put a mucilaginous protective cover over the lining of the stomach, allowing the healing processes to take place more effectively underneath.

Other digestive remedies like chamomile and lemon balm make pleasant and effective teas to reduce the inflammation. The liver may be involved, so a good bitter tonic like *gentian, especially taken before meals, will help to normalize its function. If there is a good deal of flatulence, ginger will help, or less pungent remedies like caraway or coriander if ginger is too hot. It is important to keep up a good intake of fluids such as herb teas and diluted fruit juices, even if the appetite is reduced and solid food is avoided.

CAUTION

Gentian should not be taken by people who have gastric or duodenal ulcers.

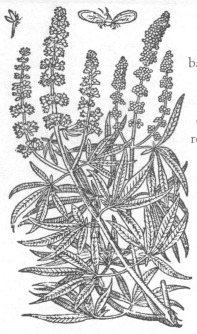

BOILS

These small local infections developing at the base of a hair shaft can be very painful if the skin is stretched tight by the swelling. Usually they will come to a head and discharge after a few days, then the skin returns to normal. If they recur it could be the sign of an underlying condition like diabetes, so professional attention should then be sought.

The herbalist's approach is to help the body in its natural way of dealing with an infection. Remedies that help the immune system, like echinacea and garlic (taken by mouth and crushed and applied to the affected area) should be taken. Then burdock and clivers will help to remove the waste products of the infection. A poultice made of slippery elm powder and chickweed can be applied over a boil to help it come to a head and discharge – this clears much of the waste products and gives the internal organs less work to do. Comfrey ointment applied after the infection has cleared will help the repair of the skin and minimize scar-formation.

CAUTION

If boils recur, seek professional advice.

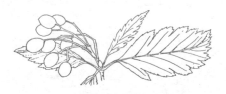

BRUISES

The one remedy that works particularly well to heal bruises in the shortest possible time is *arnica. Bruises are leakages of blood into the tissues, formed when there has been injury to the blood vessels. There is usually some degree of general swelling and inflammation as well. The best initial treatment is to soak the affected area in cold water. This helps to constrict the blood vessels, so that swelling and bruising are minimized. Then apply witch-hazel generously over the whole area to act as an astringent (again, this will reduce inflammation). When this has dried, apply arnica ointment. Arnica contains substances that help to break down the blood into its constituents, which can then be absorbed into the circulation and recycled (when a bruise turns different colours before it disappears this is due to the breakdown process).

If it seems that your skin bruises exceptionally easily, it may be due to a shortage of Vitamin C or rutin in your diet. Both of these contribute to the formation of the protein fibres in the skin and blood vessels that give them structural strength. Most fruits, particularly citrus, contain both Vitamin C and rutin. Buckwheat tea is also a good source of rutin, or it can be taken in tablet form.

CAUTION

Do not apply arnica to broken skin.

CAUTION

Do not attempt to treat any but the most minor burns by yourself.

BURNS

You should treat only minor burns yourself. If a large area of skin is broken it is a sitting target for infection, and also the site for fluid loss. The first thing to do is to soak the area in clean cold water to take the excess heat out of the skin as soon as possible. This minimizes the damage done by excess heat and avoids the development of unnecessary inflammation. When the pain has lessened, dry the area and apply witch-hazel, which will help to form a protective surface over the burn. Healing remedies like marigold, St John's wort or oil of lavender will then help. Keep the area protected with sterile dressings until the skin has healed.

For sunburn, apply generous amounts of witch-hazel to the affected area. The most effective technique is to place a lint pad or equivalent over the area and to keep this permanently moistened with witch-hazel. Pour more of it on every half an hour or so. This quickly takes away the pain and protects the damaged skin. An overnight application of wheatgerm oil or pure Vitamin E oil helps promote rapid healing.

CANDIDA INFECTION

I am limiting consideration to mouth and vaginal candida (thrush) infection only, as the possibility of generalized candida infection is a controversial matter and needs professional diagnosis. Localized candida can be diagnosed by taking swabs. The standard orthodox treatment is antifungal lozenges, pessaries or creams; although these usually work effectively at the time, they don't help to prevent a recurrence of the problem. Some women seem particularly prone to recurrences, and it is here that herbal treatment has most to offer.

There are two approaches to treatment. The first is to support the immune system, which is the body's natural defence against infection, with remedies like echinacea taken internally. Taking garlic and plain live yogurt in the diet will also help this. The second step is to use antifungal herbal remedies locally, as a mouthwash against oral thrush or as a *douche for vaginal infection. Use marigold and *thyme in the form of teas, made to twice the usual strength as you want a mouthwash rather than something to swallow. Add one quarter of a teaspoon of tincture of myrrh to about one quarter of a cup of the mouthwash, which is the amount to use for each dose. It will taste horrible, but remember that after swishing each mouthful round in your mouth and then gargling with it, you can finally spit it out.

CAUTION

Seek professional help for generalized candida infections.
Do not use a vaginal douche or take thyme during pregnancy.

The same formula can be used for vaginal thrush, but if it stings it should be watered down until it can be used without discomfort. Try applying a tiny dab to the vagina and leaving it for a few hours to check whether or not it is going to sting. If you don't have a douche you can soak a tampon in the lotion and insert it for several hours – many women have found this successful.

CATARRH AND SINUSITIS

Many people find they have trouble with catarrh that is not always due to an infection. Causes can be a damp or polluted atmosphere, allergies, or abnormalities such as polyps in the membranes lining the nose and sinus cavities. Some people find that if they eat too many milk-based foods such as cheese and yogurt they get catarrh. It can also be a sign of inadequate elimination elsewhere; for example, sluggish bowel function. Once the catarrh is produced it can easily become infected, leading to the uncomfortable or downright painful condition of sinusitis.

To treat the problem effectively it will be necessary to look at all aspects of a person's health, but the general guideline is to try a plain wholefood diet as free as possible of processed foods. Increase your intake of fruit and vegetables, which are natural cleansing foods. Allergies and polyps will probably need professional attention. You can reduce the risk of infections by taking garlic and echinacea, and by using tincture of myrrh as a gargle. Use Friar's Balsam in a *steam inhalation as well. A pleasant tea to soothe the inflamed membranes can be made from elderflower and peppermint, and a warming remedy like ginger or angelica may help if the problem is affected by cold or damp weather. The general cleansing remedies like dandelion root to help the liver and *celery seed to help the kidneys are very useful. Cudweed, golden rod and ground ivy are the most direct anticatarrhal remedies available.

There are some remedies that will help when applied externally to the affected areas: I use a lotion or oil containing *cayenne, myrrh and golden seal. Stroke this gently onto the skin over the sinuses twice a day. The cayenne will bring a feeling of warmth which most people find pleasant, but occasionally you might feel uncomfortably hot: if this happens, just dilute the lotion with more water or oil until an acceptable strength is achieved. Be careful not to get the lotion in your eyes, as it will sting, and wash it off your hands thoroughly after applying it.

C A U T I O N

Do not take celery seeds in pregnancy.
Do not apply cayenne to broken skin, and be careful not to get it in your eyes.

CHEST INFECTIONS

As the consequences of untreated chest infections can be dangerous, they should always be treated professionally. However, there are numerous remedies that will help your body deal with the infection and phlegm more effectively.

C A U T I O N

Always seek professional help if you have a chest infection.
Some people with asthma may find that steam is irritating to their chests. Steam inhalations should not be used in these cases.

Try garlic and echinacea to help you fight off the infection - in fact, garlic is one of the few treatments that helps against viruses as well as bacteria. A *steam inhalation of Friar's Balsam will take the anti-infective and soothing properties of the balsam right into the lungs where it can help rapidly. The infection will provoke inflammation in the lungs, resulting in discomfort and possibly wheezing. This can be soothed with *elecampane, white horehound, *coltsfoot, *thyme and aniseed, which all help to loosen tight phlegm so it can be coughed up more easily. A warming remedy like ginger or angelica can help too, particularly if the problem is aggravated by cold or damp weather.

CAUTION

Do not take elecampane and thyme in pregnancy.
Long-term use of coltsfoot is not advised.

CHILBLAINS AND POOR CIRCULATION

The winter weather in Britain has an adverse effect on a wide range of illnesses, but there is one that is almost exclusively due to the effects of cold, namely chilblains. These tender, itchy pink blotches develop on the parts of the body that get cold for too long, usually the feet and hands. When they are exposed to cold, the small local blood vessels in the skin constrict to minimize the amount of blood and heat flowing to the skin. The result is that inflammation develops. People vary in their susceptibility to cold: some never seem to feel it, while others have to be careful, even in the summer.

The best herbal remedies for this are those that stimulate the circulation. Most of the hot-tasting spices like cayenne and ginger will help: the sensation they produce on the tongue mirrors the action they have on the body as a whole. There is a very good traditional combination called 'Composition Essence' which is a mixture of these types of circulatory stimulants in a pleasant-tasting base, available from most health/herb shops. Take about one quarter of a teaspoon of this stirred into a hot

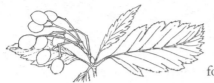

drink (it makes a delicious drink when added to hot fruit juice) several times a day. If these remedies are too fierce for your stomach, the gentler ones like angelica will still help. As well as taking them internally, the hot spices can be made into a tea and used in hand and footbaths. Be careful not to use these on broken skin, as they will sting.

The other useful group of remedies to take internally are the diaphoretics, like elderflower, yarrow and limeflowers. They help to draw the circulation of blood to the skin, thus increasing warmth.

COLDS

There is no way to avoid exposure to the thousands of rapidly mutating viruses responsible for head-colds. People's resistance to them varies enormously, and can be affected by problems like poor diet, stress, etc. If you seem to be susceptible it is worth taking the following steps to help your immune system.

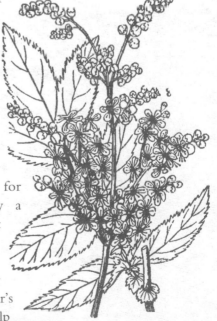

Take garlic every day as it helps against both viral and bacterial infections. Vitamin C is very important too. Ensure you have at least two pieces of fresh fruit daily, and three portions of vegetables. If you can't manage this, take a Vitamin C supplement. Many people seem to benefit from taking cod liver oil for its Vitamins A and D. Also, try a mineral supplement and make sure it contains zinc.

Once the infection has struck, take boneset, elderflower, peppermint or hyssop to calm the feverish stage. Friar's Balsam as a *steam inhalation can help with the catarrh. If you have to work through the period of the infection, Composition Essence helps to keep your alertness and concentration as sharp as possible. Try to get as much rest as you can, though, as your body's priority will be to fight the infection rather than to divert energy to any other activity.

CAUTION

Some people with asthma may find that steam is irritating to their chests. Steam inhalations should not be used in these cases.

COLIC

This intense abdominal pain is caused by the contraction of rings of muscle along the intestines. It usually occurs as a result of irritation to the membranes lining the intestines, and is part of the group of reactions by which the digestion can rid itself of dangerous substances: these contractions are an extreme form of the movement by which everything is propelled through the digestive system and then out of the body. The irritating substance can be due to infections (when diarrhoea is also likely to be present) or to foods to which the person is sensitive. Certain strong laxatives can also bring on colic; to avoid this, it is recommended that they are taken with carminative remedies. Flatulence often accompanies colic, and can be very uncomfortable in itself.

Fortunately, there are numerous palatable herbal remedies, the carminatives, that can relieve both problems. They work by soothing the lining of the digestive system and relaxing the cramping muscles. The best-known traditional combination is babies' gripe-water, which contains dill and ginger.

Other suitable remedies include chamomile, caraway, fennel seed and coriander. Some of these are ingredients in after-dinner liqueurs such as Kummel and Chartreuse, because of their pleasant taste and useful digestion-aiding properties. In the East many of the carminative seeds are customarily chewed after meals to aid the digestion.

CONSTIPATION

There can be several causes of this condition. They must be investigated before the appropriate treatment can be decided, because the use of laxative remedies is not always the best solution to the problem. To produce a normal bowel-motion, there must be a phase of contraction in the rings of muscle along the intestines, which propels the food forward, followed by a phase of relaxation in which more food is pushed forward from behind. These movements combine to form a wave of contraction passing along the length of the gut, known as peristalsis. The wave needs to be continuous to work properly, so if some of the muscular contractions get out of phase the result is that the food is no longer efficiently pushed through.

This can be due to the muscles being sluggish and underactive, or to them being too tense and not relaxing properly. Another possibility is that the food going through is not soft enough for the muscles to work on. Your first consideration should be to rule out this possibility by changing your diet. In the recent past it has been suggested that bran be added to the diet to increase fibre. Many people find bran quite irritating, though, so I think an increase in fruit, vegetables and wholegrain cereals generally is likely to be better tolerated. Try adding prunes or figs to your breakfast cereal, which should be wholewheat or oats. Make sure you eat wholemeal bread rather than white. Have plenty of fluids to drink through the day - about three to four pints in total.

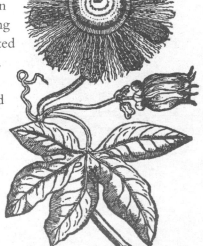

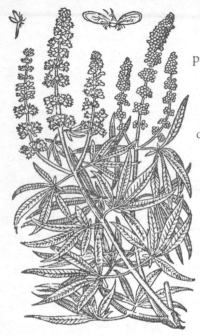

If the stool is still hard, try a softening agent like psyllium seeds. These form a gel when you mix them with water, helping to keep everything soft as they go through your insides. If these steps don't help and you have a very sluggish digestion, the next remedy to try is *cascara. This is available as the crude bark, or in several pharmaceutical preparations from the chemist shop. Cascara may occasionally cause discomfort – it works by irritating the upper intestine, which provokes a reflex increase in bowel activity about eight hours later – so it is best to take a carminative remedy like ginger or caraway with it. The most famous laxative, *senna, has a stronger action still, and the pods should be taken with carminatives in small doses only to start with: try one quarter to one half of a teaspoon of the crushed pods, once or twice a day. Senna is also available in tablet form, where the suggested dosage will be written on the pack.

If your abdomen has a very tense feeling, or if the constipation is due to nervous tension, these laxatives should be avoided and instead the relaxing digestive remedies, such as chamomile or lemon balm, should be taken along with the psyllium seeds. Try getting more brisk exercise, and massage your abdomen, working in a circular motion starting low down on the right side, up to and across the solar plexus area and downwards on the left side. This can help relieve pockets of tension.

C A U T I O N

*Cascara and senna should not be used during pregnancy.
If the constipation needs treatment for longer than ten days, consult a professional.*

COUGHS

Coughing is part of the normal response of the lungs to any source of irritation. This can be due to several possible causes, which may require different approaches to treatment. Chest infections, allergic reactions, cold damp weather, air pollution and asthma can all cause a cough. When the membranes lining the airways are irritated, they produce mucus (phlegm) to form a protective covering, and also to engulf the

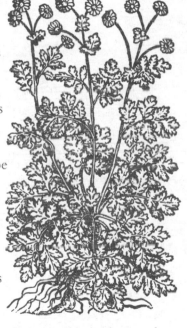

source of the irritation if it is harmful bacteria or particles of pollution. This mucus is then wafted up out of the deep parts of the lungs by the movement of tiny hairs, and when it enters the main airways the act of coughing expels it into the mouth.

Thus coughing functions to keep the lungs cleansed of harmful substances, and the herbalist will seek to support and ease it rather than suppress it. The underlying cause must be treated, and in addition remedies that help to soothe the lining of the lungs, and keep the phlegm very liquid and easy to cough up, will be chosen. *Elecampane, white horehound and *coltsfoot are ideal for this job. Although the cough may seem unpleasant, providing it is not painful or unproductive of phlegm it is doing vital work to restore health. When the cause of the irritation has subsided, the herbal remedies will help the cough to calm down. The undesirable type of cough is the very dry, painful, unproductive type. The same remedies will help encourage the production of mucus, which will ease a dry cough. Add *thyme which also helps to loosen mucus, and use a *steam inhalation with Friars' Balsam – the warm steam will have a loosening effect.

CAUTION

Elecampane and thyme should not be taken during pregnancy.
Long-term use of coltsfoot is not advised.
If asthma is suspected, consult a professional.
Some people with asthma may find that steam is irritating to their chests.
Steam inhalations should not be used in these cases.

CUTS AND GRAZES

The first step is to stop any blood loss by applying pressure over the area of the minor wound with a clean pad of lint, etc. For a small wound witch-hazel will help stop the blood and reduce the surrounding swelling. Then ensure that the area is clean: dilute a teaspoon of tincture of myrrh in 150ml (¼ pint) of sterile water and bathe the skin with this. It might sting, but it is an excellent antiseptic remedy. Cover with a clean dressing, and when a scab has formed a healing ointment can be applied to speed up the process of repair. Try marigold or St John's wort, which are also good anti-inflammatory remedies, or comfrey, which helps to speed healing and has a reputation for reducing the risk of scar formation.

CYSTITIS

This can be due to an *infection or a chill, or with some people it can occur if too much of the wrong type of food is eaten. The symptoms vary: there can be pain in the lower abdomen, pain when passing water, or frequent urges to pass water. Rest and warmth are needed in all cases, and a high fluid intake (about 2.25 litres/4 pints total a day) is required to keep the urine dilute, as a high concentration of any waste products in it is likely to add to the discomfort. An infection will need professional assessment, as the kidneys will be vulnerable if it spreads.

*Bearberry is the most useful auxiliary remedy to help clear urinary infections. If the problem is due to a chill or food sensitivity, soothing remedies like *horsetail are excellent. A diuretic such as dandelion leaf will ensure the production of plenty of urine.

If recurrent infections are a problem, take a glass of cranberry juice every day. This helps to prevent the bacteria from latching on to the lining of the bladder and results in them being flushed out of the bladder before they have a chance to multiply.

C A U T I O N

Seek professional help if you suspect a vaginal infection.
Bearberry should not be taken in pregnancy, or by people
with kidney problems.
Horsetail should not be taken by people with heart problems.

DANDRUFF

This is a type of inflammation of the scalp, associated with the production of flaking skin. It involves malfunctioning of the glands that produce oil in the scalp, and the skin on the scalp can be either very dry or very oily. It can also be extremely tender. The herbalist will use the 'cleansing' remedies internally, the same as would be used for other skin problems like eczema. In addition, lotions can be used to help correct the oil production. If the scalp is very oily, strong teas of nettles, rosemary and witch-hazel can be applied. Dry scalps may respond better to a lotion of nettles and chamomile. Apply the lotions directly to the scalp, regularly. For mild cases it may be enough to add them to the final rinsing water when the hair is washed.

DEBILITY

Many people nowadays feel permanently below par, as a result of the hectic lives they lead. Anti-stress techniques include physical exercise, yoga and meditation. Nervine remedies that help to nourish and support the function of the nervous system include damiana and *ginseng. It is normal to feel lacking in strength and vitality when convalescing after an acute illness. Remember that rest is the natural requirement during convalescence to enable the body to return to normal functioning. Wood betony and vervain are both good general convalescent tonics. *Gentian will help restore the appetite and digestion to normal. Take oats in the diet, as porridge, oatcakes or flapjacks: they are a particularly nourishing cereal.

CAUTION

Do not take ginseng in pregnancy or if you have high blood pressure. It should not be taken with other stimulants (such as coffee), or for more than a month at a time.

Gentian is not suitable for people with gastric or duodenal ulcers.

DEPRESSION

This term covers a wide degree of emotional and physical reactions, and the underlying cause must be discovered. It is often beneficial to see a counsellor or psychotherapist to work through this. What herbal medicine can offer is a treatment to help with the physical side of the problem: the remedies for debility can help to support the normal function and nutritional tone of the nerves, enabling the sufferer to cope better with

stressful or painful emotions. If other aspects of
physical functioning are affected, like digestive
or sleep disturbances, they can be treated with suitable
remedies. It is worth keeping to a plan of
exercise to keep the body ticking over healthily.
This is probably the last thing a depressed person
feels like doing, but it can bring a welcome
feeling of wellbeing afterwards.

DIARRHOEA

As with most functions of the body, the
frequency of normal bowel-motions varies. If
the stool is also very loose and watery, and
discomfort or colic is present, it can be classed as
being in need of treatment. There are several
possible causes of this type of problem, and the
appropriate treatment will be different for each one.

The first thing to consider is whether or not the reaction may be due to
an infection in the digestive system. A speeding up of the elimination of
harmful organisms is a very useful, though uncomfortable, mechanism to
reduce the duration of the infection. The same mechanism works against
certain foods that may have an irritating effect on some people, and also
against *poisonous or irritant substances that have been consumed.

CAUTION

If poisoning is suspected call the emergency services straight away.

For an infection, take garlic to help clear it. Plain live yogurt is also a
soothing anti-infective food. The intensity of the elimination reaction can
be calmed with agrimony, which is a good astringent, reducing
inflammation in the lining of the digestive tract. Mucilaginous remedies
like marshmallow root and slippery elm powder help by having a direct

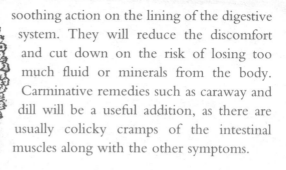

soothing action on the lining of the digestive system. They will reduce the discomfort and cut down on the risk of losing too much fluid or minerals from the body. Carminative remedies such as caraway and dill will be a useful addition, as there are usually colicky cramps of the intestinal muscles along with the other symptoms.

DYSPEPSIA

Numerous disturbances of the digestion come under this heading. The mildest symptoms are flatulence and discomfort, which may develop into indigestion and heartburn (these are both associated with too much stomach acid, and may precede the more serious problem of ulcers).

CAUTION

If the dyspepsia doesn't clear up quickly, consult a professional.

The diet is the first thing to look at. Cut out any foods you suspect of causing problems. Consider particularly rich, fatty, sweet, highly fibrous, spicy or overlarge meals ('small and often' suits most people much better). Keep to a plain and fairly bland diet until you feel an improvement.

The following herbal remedies will all be helpful in calming the disturbances. Carminatives like caraway and fennel are very useful for reducing flatulence and colic. Chamomile acts as a good soothing remedy to reduce inflammation in the stomach. Meadowsweet helps to counteract too much acid and supports normal stomach functioning. Marshmallow and slippery elm powder soothe the stomach by forming a protective lining of mucus over the inflamed surface. *Liquorice also helps the formation of a resistant mucus cover on any damaged area, and helps the healing of underlying erosions or ulcers. You have plenty of remedies to choose from, so pick those that seem most appropriate to your particular symptoms.

C A U T I O N

Do not take liquorice in pregnancy.

ECZEMA

This is one of the most frequent problems I deal with, and one of the most difficult! Although in orthodox medicine eczema is considered to be one condition, I have found it to have so many possible causes that it needs a more detailed assessment than just about any other disease. The more accurate observations that can be made about its causes, the better the chance of finding a successful treatment.

Most people with eczema tend to have a dry skin. This can cause discomfort and irritation in itself, as a skin that has less oil than normal is more easily damaged by cold winds, contact with detergents, etc. When it becomes inflamed as well as dry this is classed as eczema. The inflammation can develop as a result of allergic reactions, such as to pollen, chemicals or foods (eczema and asthma of allergic origin are often seen in the same person or family), or it can be due to nervous stress.

If allergies are suspected, I think a consultation with a professional is advisable to plan an approach to investigating what the causes might be. If the eczema is generally calm but flares up periodically it will be easier to pinpoint the causes, but if it is a constant problem an elimination diet may be necessary – see entry for Allergies. One suggestion I have for all eczema sufferers is to cut out all cows' milk products (milk, cheese, yogurt and processed foods that contain whey or casein) for one month, replacing them with soya milk, goats' or sheep's milk cheese, soya yogurt, etc. With about 10 per cent of sufferers, I have found that if they do this the problem clears spontaneously and there is rarely the need for any other treatment. The self-discipline involved in the diet is well repaid by the improvement it brings for these people. For those who don't benefit, at least the possibility of cows' milk allergy has been ruled out. If contact allergies are detected, the offending substances must be avoided as far as possible to give the skin a chance to heal. Stress can be counteracted with herbal remedies such as chamomile, limeflowers and lemon balm, or the more potent ★passion flower and valerian.

There are few remedies that are applicable to all cases of eczema, but the 'cleansers' such as clivers and red clover, dandelion root and nettles are all worth trying. These help to improve functions such as liver, kidney and lymphatic system activity. The list of remedies that have helped eczema sufferers seems endless, but this is because individual people respond differently to various lines of treatment: there is no such thing as a standard prescription for this problem.

External applications can bring relief from the irritation and can help to moisturize the skin. Chickweed ointment has the best reputation for reducing itching and inflammation. Marigold and chamomile ointments and pure Vitamin E oil are also well worth trying.

CAUTION

Do not take passion flower in pregnancy.

EYE IRRITATION

When the eyes are feeling sore, bloodshot, watery or itchy they have been irritated by something, which must be identified. Some people's eyes are much more sensitive than others and may water as a reaction to wind or cold weather exposure.

> ### CAUTION
> *If an eye infection is suspected you should get professional advice.*

Irritation can be caused by allergies and airborne pollutants such as smoke or chemical fumes. The best herbal remedy to calm the irritation is the aptly named eyebright. This is an astringent particularly suited to use on the surface of the eye. It does not get rid of an *infection (which will need its own treatment) but will help to calm the resulting discomfort. Many people find that bathing the eyes with eyebright is a successful way to deal with allergic irritation, and it is certainly very effective in helping recovery from exposure to irritating pollutants. Follow exactly the directions given in Chapter 6 (Eyebright entry) for preparing the eyebath, as this will ensure that the preparation is sterile. An enhanced action against infections will be achieved by adding golden seal to the eyebright.

FEVER

> ### CAUTION
> *If the symptoms accompanying the fever are severe the problem may need professional attention.*

A mild fever accompanying a head-cold can be treated with a range of herbal remedies. In the initial stages, when the fever is building up, you will probably feel shivery and cold – the body is conserving heat to create an environment that is hostile to the infecting organism. You can add to the success of this by taking stimulating remedies such as cayenne, ginger or the traditional combination known as Composition Essence. This can be bought from most health/herb shops. It is a spicy tasting mixture of remedies including cayenne and cinnamon that have a warming, stimulating effect on the circulation. You will need about a quarter to a half teaspoon dose at a time, added to a hot drink – it makes a delicious drink with hot fruit juice. When the feeling of fever becomes noticeable, the temperature can be regulated by taking the diaphoretic remedies that promote perspiration. Boneset, yarrow, elderflower and limeflowers all have this action. After recovering from a fever, most people have a poor appetite and feel lacking in energy for some time. Bitter tonics like *gentian will help the appetite, and general convalescent tonics such as vervain are also helpful.

CAUTION

Gentian should not be taken by people who have gastric or duodenal ulcers.

GUM AND MOUTH ULCERS

These are small, intensely painful erosions of the membranes in the mouth. Some people seem to be prone to having them frequently; in others these ulcers indicate that the person is run down – possibly after an infection, or as a result of lack of sleep, stress, poor diet, etc. These possibilities need considering to see if there is a way the health can be improved generally. Remedies to help internal cleansing, like burdock, dandelion root, echinacea and clivers, will be helpful. A good local application is tincture of myrrh, which can be diluted and used as a mouthwash for an extensive problem or dabbed neat onto the individual ulcer. This will sting for a second but soon wears off, after which the ulcer heals much more quickly.

HAEMORRHOIDS

A huge number of people suffer from these swellings around the back passage, which vary in the degree of discomfort they cause. Some can be almost symptomless, while others are itchy, tender or extremely painful. Some cause loss of blood, most commonly a few spots occurring after a bowel evacuation. More often called piles, they occur when the veins around the back passage become dilated and varicosed, with the result that blood tends to 'pool' in them instead of being efficiently transported on its way back to the heart. They are usually caused by an increase in pressure within the abdomen (such as during pregnancy or during bowel disturbances – either constipation or diarrhoea can provoke the problem). The extra pressure, added to the downwards pressure of gravity, overcomes the upwards pressure of the healthy circulation pushing the blood onwards. Then the walls of the veins stretch too much and lose their elasticity, resulting in the swelling.

The first line of treatment is to reduce the extra pressure if this is due to abnormal bowel function – see under Diarrhoea or Constipation. Other remedies for internal use are those that help the condition of the blood vessels, so try yarrow and hawthorn. Include dandelion root to help with liver function, as blood from the haemorrhoids drains back through the liver before reaching the main circulation. Apply a lotion made of a strong tea of lesser celandine mixed with witch-hazel to the swellings to help shrink them, and use a lotion or cream containing chamomile if they are itchy or inflamed.

HANGOVERS

I include this on the basis that even the most health-conscious person might overconsume alcohol at times. The rate at which alcohol is normally broken down by the liver is about one unit (275ml/½ pint of beer, one glass of wine or a single measure of a spirit) per hour, though individuals will of course vary. If you restrict your intake to about this amount, and take plenty of non-alcoholic drinks in between (which is often the easiest way to reduce your overall consumption of alcohol), you shouldn't have too many problems the next day. But if you do overdo it, you need to take plenty of water or diluted fruit juices to replace lost fluid, and some liver-stimulating remedies to speed up the breaking down of the last of the alcohol in your system. Try dandelion root, *gentian or *hops. These will all taste very bitter, but put up with that as it is the bitter taste that stimulates the body's recovery. Other problems may include general digestive discomfort, as a result of the irritating effect alcohol can have on the lining of the gut: take chamomile, lemon balm or peppermint tea for this.

CAUTION

Gentian should not be taken by people who have gastric or duodenal ulcers. Hops are not suitable for people suffering from depression.

HEADACHES AND MIGRAINE

There are numerous causes of these problems, and it may be necessary to get professional help for some of them. The most common problem is the occasional stress or tiredness headache. The best remedies for these are the gentle relaxing herbs like chamomile, limeflowers and wood betony. More persistent headaches will be helped by the regular inclusion of these in the diet, plus other stress-reducing activities like physical exercise, yoga and meditation. Headaches connected with tension in the neck muscles will benefit from massage around that area with an oil or lotion made from lavender, cramp bark and *cayenne.

Migraines can be triggered by many things: bright light, particular foods, skipping a meal and certain smells have all been known to cause problems. Try to track down the triggers in each case, as you have a much better chance of reducing the frequency if you can avoid these. The most effective herbal remedy to take long term to avoid the attacks is *feverfew, which seems to help the problem for about 70 per cent of sufferers. It is most helpful for people who describe the pain as a 'cold' feeling that is relieved by a warming application to the area. You may have to take feverfew for several months before getting the full benefit, so be patient. While the headaches are still occurring, take the remedies suggested for stress headaches, or try yarrow, which helps to correct the circulatory disturbance thought to be the mechanism behind the problem.

Dandelion root or *gentian both help to stimulate liver function, and this approach often proves successful with headaches that have no other apparent cause.

C A U T I O N

Consult a professional if headaches are persistent or recur frequently.
Be careful not to get cayenne in your eyes. Do not apply to broken skin.
Feverfew is not suitable for use in pregnancy.
Gentian should not be taken by people who have gastric
or duodenal ulcers.

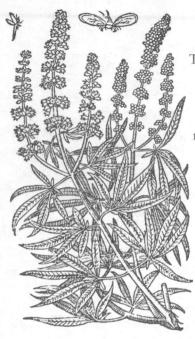

HEART DISEASE

This is of course a problem requiring professional management, but there are plenty of foods and herbal remedies that will help prevent the diseases developing and that can play a useful role in a recovery programme. There are several aspects of heart disease that give rise to differing symptoms, but the underlying causes are all very similar.

As we get older, small changes occur in the walls of the arteries, causing them to narrow somewhat. The patches causing this are called atheromas and are a natural feature of the ageing process. Problems start to occur when the atheromas attract cholesterol and other fats which accumulate and produce a plaque. These plaques can then attract calcium, making the artery harder and less elastic. This is known as atherosclerosis or, more popularly, hardening of the arteries.

CAUTION

Seek professional help immediately if heart problems are suspected.

Further complications set in when the plaques become larger and start to restrict the flow of blood to the organs or tissues. Restriction of the blood flow to the heart can leave it short of oxygen, especially when the body's oxygen demand increases during exercise or stress. The pain experienced when the heart is starved of oxygen is called angina pectoris.

Blood pressure may become raised, posing a further risk to the condition of the arteries. The plaques may cause damage to the arteries and these damaged areas may be the focus for the formation of a blood clot. This can completely block the artery - this is what happens in a heart-attack, when one of the arteries carrying blood to the heart muscle becomes blocked. The muscle cells cannot survive without blood, and some portion of the heart muscle may die and be replaced by scar tissue. The severity of the symptoms and consequences will depend on how large an area of heart muscle has been affected.

It is thought that many of these problems are caused by eating too much fatty foods and not getting enough exercise – see Chapter 3 for more about this. General advice is to cut down on fats, especially from animal sources such as butter and lard, and remove obvious fat from meat like bacon and chops. Avoid processed meats such as sausages and burgers because the fat is mixed in with the meat and so you can't remove it. Eggs and cheese are also rich in fats – don't have more than two or three eggs a week or 110g (¼lb) of cheese. Where possible, choose low fat dairy products like cottage cheese and fromage frais. Ordinary margarine is little better than butter, as the processing technique turns the vegetable fat in it into a similar form to animal fat. Use a low-fat spread instead. Choose lean poultry and oily fish such as mackerel, salmon, sardines, etc.: the type of fats they contain, unlike meat fats, are positively beneficial to your health.

Good quality olive oil (unfortunately quite expensive, but think of it as a healthy substitute for the expensive meats that you could be buying less of in future) has been shown in clinical trials to be the most beneficial oil to use. Cut down on tea and coffee: the caffeine in them can cause stress responses that may affect the heart. Try coffee alternatives like chicory or dandelion root – the flavours are different from coffee but very pleasant when you are used to them.

Foods that are positively beneficial, and can be taken in unlimited amounts, are as follows. Onions, garlic and shallots help to reduce the clotting tendencies of the blood. Oatbran, beans and pulses, grapefruit (the whole fruit, not just the juice), oranges, apples, strawberries, bananas, carrots and aubergines all help to reduce harmful cholesterol. If you have a diet that includes a wide range of fruit and vegetables you can't go too far wrong, as it is quite possible that further research will reveal they provide benefits as yet unknown.

Herbal remedies that are compatible with orthodox medication for problems like angina, high blood pressure or thrombosis are hawthorn berries, *motherwort, limeflowers, yarrow and ginger. These all have a supportive, nourishing effect on the heart and blood vessels that will strengthen the tissues without affecting the rate or rhythm of the heart.

C A U T I O N

Do not take motherwort in the first eight months of pregnancy.

I N F L U E N Z A

For details on the natural treatment of this problem, see the entries for Colds and Chest infections. Bear in mind that 'flu can be much more debilitating and take longer to recover from than those conditions, so try to get plenty of rest during the convalescent stage. Convalescent remedies to restore energy and vigour include vervain and white horehound (which is particularly useful if there is a problem with a residual cough). *Gentian root is excellent specifically for restoring the appetite to normal. Follow a plain diet with plenty of fresh fruit and vegetables while you are convalescing – these supply the body's needs for vitamins and minerals without being too demanding on the digestion.

C A U T I O N

Gentian should not be taken by people who have gastric or duodenal ulcers.

INSECT BITES & STINGS

For minor problems where the skin has been broken, an application of tincture of myrrh is advisable to prevent infections developing. This will sting for a moment if it is applied neat, but is worth the short time of discomfort because it also seems to help promote the healing of the injury. Some people react very dramatically to bites, and may find that as well as the myrrh an application of witch-hazel reduces the swelling and itching. If a large area becomes affected it may be slow to heal – try comfrey or chickweed ointment to improve this. If this problem happens regularly throughout the summer, try taking a combination of remedies regularly to reduce the reaction: burdock, clivers, dandelion root, nettles and red clover may all help to calm the inflammatory tendency of the skin.

For *stings, apply a soothing remedy like chickweed, marigold or St John's wort to the affected area.

CAUTION

Allergic reactions to stings can be very serious, so seek professional help immediately if any breathing difficulties develop.

INSOMNIA

This can be a manifestation of a general state of nervous tension, or it can result from a period of disturbed sleep routine, as seen sometimes in people who have to change between day and night work shifts. The first remedies to try are the relaxing herbal teas like limeflower and chamomile. These

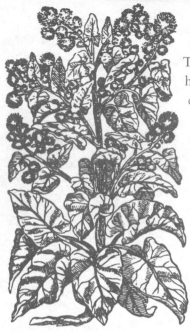

will both help to ease tension and thus enable normal sleep to occur more readily. Try them for a week or so. If you are still having problems, there are several commercially produced combination teas that may help. These will contain a wider range of remedies and may not be as pleasant-tasting as the previous two, but should have a more potent relaxing effect. As an alternative to these you can try the various combinations of relaxing herbal remedies marketed in tablet form. *Passion flower and valerian are two very reliable and effective relaxing remedies that are available in several formulations.

CAUTION

Do not take passion flower during pregnancy.

MENOPAUSAL PROBLEMS

At around the age of fifty most women find that their normal monthly cycle is starting to change. With some, their periods just stop and they have no other problems. Usually, though, some sort of accompanying disturbance occurs as a result of fluctuating hormone levels. These will eventually settle down at a level lower than before the menopause and should then no longer cause any problems. It is very hard to predict for individuals how long this settling down will take, however. The three herbal remedies that are useful in just about all problems connected with the menopause are agnus-castus, *motherwort and St John's wort. These can safely be taken for the duration of the disturbances.

CAUTION

Do not take motherwort, red sage or raspberry leaves if you may be pregnant rather than starting the menopause.

The most frequent problem is hot flushes, which are due to a disturbance in the circulation caused by the hormone changes. As well as motherwort and agnus-castus, try *red sage to help with this. It is fairly common to feel anxiety or panics with the flushes: if this happens, take St John's wort, chamomile or limeflowers.

Fluid retention is best treated with dandelion leaves. Irregular or heavy bleeding can be a very distressing problem. Black haw and *raspberry leaves may help with this, though I would suggest a professional consultation as there are more remedies that will help that are beyond the scope of this book. Tiredness can be alleviated with damiana.

MENSTRUAL PROBLEMS

Herbal remedies can be very successful in treating several different menstrual problems. The most useful remedy is *motherwort, which can be taken for any problem involving the womb – it has a toning and nourishing action on the female reproductive system generally. Mix other remedies with it as appropriate.

Premenstrual syndrome can cause irritability, clumsiness, poor concentration, insomnia, breast tenderness and fluid retention in the abdomen. The most useful remedy is agnus-castus, which helps the vast majority of women. It is thought to work by stabilizing fluctuations in the levels of hormones produced by the pituitary gland and ovaries. As well as this, irritability and poor concentration can be reduced by taking relaxing nervine remedies like scullcap and wood betony. Fluid retention is best dealt with by dandelion leaf, or one of the several commercial herbal combinations available from herb/health shops for this purpose.

It is important to have the correct amount of the minerals calcium and magnesium in your diet. Many women have found dietary supplements containing them to be very helpful. The required amounts are 400mg calcium and 200mg magnesium. Vitamin E is essential and may be required in supplemental doses.

For cramping pain experienced during a period try chamomile, *raspberry leaf or black haw, with a little ginger to help the circulation. Black haw is also useful to reduce heavy blood loss.

CAUTION

Do not take motherwort or raspberry leaves if you may be pregnant.

MIGRAINE
see Headaches & Migraine

MOUTH ULCERS
see Gum & Mouth Ulcers

MUSCULAR ACHES & PAINS

There can be several causes of this problem. When people start new programmes of exercise or do physical work to which they are unaccustomed it is usual to feel aches and pains for the following day or two. *If they last for longer, there may have been an injury, such as muscle fibres being torn rather than just inflamed. The way to avoid this is to start gradually and build up the duration and intensity of work over a period of time. Do

warm-up exercises involving stretches
and movements before you start -
this applies as much to the first day
of the year you spend gardening as it
does to jogging, etc. After exercise
keep the muscles warm: a relaxing
bath is an excellent idea.
Rosemary is a pleasant and
invigorating remedy to add to
the water in the form of a strong
tea. Many people find that a tablespoon of

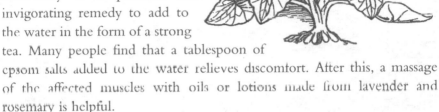

epsom salts added to the water relieves discomfort. After this, a massage
of the affected muscles with oils or lotions made from lavender and
rosemary is helpful.

C A U T I O N

Seek professional help if muscular pains persist.

If the pain is severe or longer lasting and it seems that muscles have been
injured, rest them if you can and use an oil or lotion containing some
*cayenne to improve the local circulation, and comfrey to promote the
speed of repair of the tissues. Take *celery seeds and nettles internally to help
the body clear itself of the substances produced during the inflammation.

C A U T I O N

*Do not use cayenne on broken skin and avoid it coming into contact
with the eyes.
Do not take celery seeds in pregnancy.*

PRURITIS

This problem is characterized by intense itching, and although no other signs of disease may be present, for some people it can become an intolerable problem. It often develops in areas where the skin is permanently covered by clothing and therefore warm and moist. The possibility of an *infection must be considered if the irritation is around the vagina or back passage - see the entry for Candida. Other infections will require professional diagnosis. You can cut down on the risk of infections developing by swabbing the affected area with dilute tincture of myrrh. The best anti-itching skin remedy is chickweed. Try either the ointment or, if the oil in this adds to the feeling of irritation, make a strong tea and use it as a lotion. You can also try chamomile in the same two formulations, while witch-hazel may help as an astringent application. Try using these remedies two or three times a day, although if they bring relief you can use them as frequently as you choose - they don't have side-effects so there is no need to limit the frequency of their use.

CAUTION

Seek professional advice for any suspected infection.

PSORIASIS

This widespread skin problem can come and go quite mysteriously, and there are few remedies that can be relied on to help in all cases. Like eczema, it requires a good deal of detective work on the part of the sufferer to pinpoint what factors seem to influence its course: the more that can be identified, the better the chances of treating the problem successfully. The herbalist's basic approach is to support the elimination functions of the body with remedies for the liver like dandelion root and yellow dock, while the lymphatic system and kidneys can be helped by clivers. There is often a component of stress reaction in the problem, and nervine remedies such as wood betony and *passion flower may play an important role in successful treatment. Allergies may be involved, and other problems like poor circulation or digestion, etc. must be taken into account: they can have a great effect on the problem. Try the soothing, healing remedies like chickweed, marigold, chamomile and St John's wort as ointments applied to the affected areas.

C A U T I O N

Do not take passion flower during pregnancy.

RHEUMATISM *see Arthritis & Rheumatism*

SINUSITIS *see Catarrh & Sinusitis*

SPRAINS

These injuries involve damage to the tissues around a joint, where ligaments and muscles may be torn. There is much pain and swelling around the area, and it may be difficult to tell the difference between a bad sprain and a *fractured bone.

C A U T I O N

If in doubt, seek professional attention: an X-ray may be needed to confirm the diagnosis.

For a minor sprain, apply an ice-pack or soak the area in cold water to minimize the swelling and inflammation. After this, apply witch-hazel liberally as the astringent action will be soothing and anti-inflammatory. The best remedy to speed up the healing of the injury is comfrey ointment, applied twice daily until the joint feels normal again. If any bruising is apparent, apply *arnica ointment as well to disperse this as quickly as possible.

C A U T I O N

Do not apply arnica if the skin is broken.

STRESS *see Anxiety*

SUNBURN *see Burns*

THROAT INFECTIONS

These can herald the start of a general respiratory infection, or they can be a recurrent problem in themselves for some people. The herbalist's approach is similar to that for other respiratory infections - see the entry for Colds - with a few extra remedies specifically for helping the throat area. The most important of these is *red sage, which has both a soothing astringent action and helps to fight off the infection. *Raspberry leaves are another good astringent. Take both of these as a tea, and use tincture of myrrh as a gargle two or three times a day. Prepare this by adding half a teaspoon of the tincture to a tablespoon of warm water. You can also swallow a few sips of this at the end of the gargle, as it will help the body to fight off the infection when taken internally. If the tonsils are infected take clivers as well to help the lymphatic system function as it should to fight the infection.

Recurrent sore throats are most successfully treated by taking remedies regularly for a month or so, even when the infections are not present. This gives the body the chance to build up its defences and fight off the infections when they do attack. Take echinacea and garlic every day, and make sure you have plenty of fruit and salads to get enough Vitamin C. Try the tincture of myrrh gargle once a day to ward off infections.

CAUTION

Do not take red sage in pregnancy.
Do not take raspberry leaves in the first eight months of pregnancy.

THRUSH

see Candida Infections

TOOTHACHE

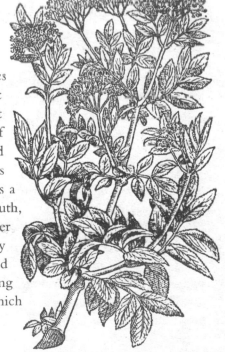

The need to use emergency remedies may arise if you can't get to see a dentist immediately. The traditional treatment for toothache is one drop of oil of cloves added to a teaspoonful of almond or olive oil, massaged into the gums around the problem tooth. This causes a very strong taste of cloves in the mouth, but does help to ease the pain. The other remedy that can help to reduce any infection is tincture of myrrh, applied neat to the gums. It has a strong astringent effect when used like this, which can reduce discomfort or pain.

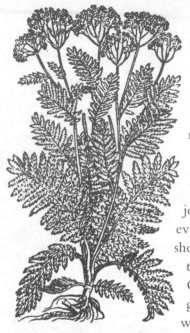

TRAVEL SICKNESS

The pleasure of travelling can be ruined for people who are subject to this problem, where pitching and rolling movements disorientate the sense of balance. Giddiness, nausea, vomiting and possible faintness are the resulting symptoms. The most useful remedy to avert these problems is ginger. This can be taken on the morning of the journey, either as a tea, tablets or capsules, or even as crystallized ginger. Small amounts should also be consumed regularly throughout the journey, at intervals of about two hours. Other remedies which can be helpful are general relaxants, such as *passion flower, which are worth taking from the night before the journey, and those that have a specific action on the digestion, like chamomile and peppermint.

CAUTION

Do not take passion flower in pregnancy.

URINARY PROBLEMS *see also Cystitis*

Most disturbances of the urinary system require professional attention, because of the vital function the kidneys perform in removing waste products from the blood and balancing fluid levels in the body. The remedies recommended here can help to restore normal function alongside other prescribed medication. In cases of infection or other inflammation such as prostate problems there is usually a good deal of very unpleasant discomfort. This can be eased with *horsetail and cornsilk. If there is an infection *bearberry is the best remedy to use.

C A U T I O N

Seek professional help for any urinary problems.
Do not take horsetail if you have a heart problem.
Bearberry should not be taken in pregnancy, or by people
with kidney problems.

In problems where there is fluid retention, which is often indicated by swelling developing in the ankles over the course of the day, dandelion leaves are the most reliable and effective remedy to help the kidneys expel the fluid. They also restore the minerals that can be lost from the body when orthodox diuretics are used.

VARICOSE VEINS

This problem occurs most commonly in the legs, where the blood has to be pushed upwards through the veins to return to the heart. The force of gravity is always working to oppose the upwards flow, and if any extra downwards pressure develops in the abdomen this can cause the veins to lose their elasticity and become dilated. They are then less efficient at conducting the blood upwards and may ache and cause fluid retention in the ankles. People who are most susceptible to these problems developing are those whose work requires them to stand still for long periods of time: they do not get the movement in their leg muscles that helps keep the circulation going. Also, pregnancy and constipation can increase downward-directed abdominal pressure. The following suggestions will help to reduce this.

1. Place a small wooden cube about

3-5cm (1-2in) high at each side of your bed at the foot end. This will create a slight slope, with your feet higher than your head, enabling gravity to return the blood from your legs to your heart more easily when you are lying down. The slope is too slight to make you feel uncomfortable.

2. When sitting still for any length of time, make your leg muscles work

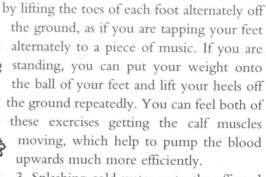

by lifting the toes of each foot alternately off the ground, as if you are tapping your feet alternately to a piece of music. If you are standing, you can put your weight onto the ball of your feet and lift your heels off the ground repeatedly. You can feel both of these exercises getting the calf muscles moving, which help to pump the blood upwards much more efficiently.

3. Splashing cold water onto the affected veins can reduce the dilation and aching, particularly in hot weather when the problem is usually at its worst.

Herbal remedies can help to some extent, though I would not claim that they can cure the problem. Try hawthorn berries and yarrow taken internally for the general benefit they bring to circulatory problems. ★Golden seal has been credited with the specific ability to help improve circulation through the veins. Externally, apply marigold and witch-hazel regularly to reduce the dilation and discomfort.

CAUTION

Do not take golden seal in pregnancy.

Rutin is a vitamin-related substance which can be taken as a supplement. Along with Vitamin C, it plays an important part in the formation of strong protein fibres in the skin and blood vessels. Rutin is one of a group of substances known as the bioflavonoids which are now added to many Vitamin C supplements. Lemon juice is a good natural source of them.

WARTS AND VERRUCAE

These unsightly hard growths on the skin can be caused by a virus, particularly verrucae which are easily picked up at places such as swimming pools. They can be painful if they occur on areas like the soles of the feet that take a lot of pressure. The most successful herbal remedy for clearing them is greater celandine. The fresh juice is needed, and enough for one application is obtained by picking one stem of the plant and using the drop of juice that appears at the end. simply dab it onto the wart and let it dry. Do this twice a day until the wart has gone (this will take about two weeks). The juice is a bright yellow colour, but turns brown when it has dried on the skin: the area is rather conspicuous for the duration of the treatment, so try to avoid getting it on the surrounding skin. However, balanced against this is the benefit that there are no side-effects and no discomfort involved. I have used this treatment several times on my young son and other children, and have found it to be free of problems.

You may wonder where to obtain the fresh plant to start with. Find a wild flower guide and check to see what it looks like: it is a common weed in many places, growing even in city areas. The seed pods produced from summer onwards will give numerous plants the following year. Otherwise, some specialist nurseries have it for sale, as some of the double-flowered varieties are very attractive. They are just as effective as the wild type.

PREGNANCY, BIRTH AND CHILDHOOD PROBLEMS

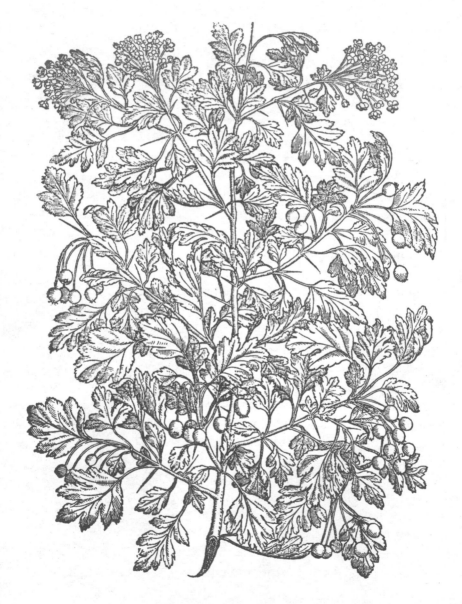

HERBS FOR PREGNANCY & BIRTH

The gentle nature of herbal remedies makes them very well suited for use when the risk of side-effects from an orthodox treatment is of particular concern. Problems occurring during pregnancy or childhood require an exceptionally safe approach to treatment.

If you have looked through Chapter 6 (the alphabetical guide to the remedies) you will have noticed warnings that some herbs should not be used during pregnancy. Herbalists always have the highest standards of safety in mind, and though these remedies are generally quite free from side-effects, the special circumstances of pregnancy require extra caution in the use of some of them. The first three months of pregnancy are crucial to the development of the baby and it would be best if no medicines at all were taken during this time. This concern of course applies to all other substances a pregnant woman might consume, including alcohol and cigarettes. There are two reasons for caution: some remedies may have an effect on the development of the baby and some may trigger contractions of the womb that could result in a premature labour. I don't know of any cases where this has actually happened after herbal remedies have been taken, but practitioners will err on the side of caution in this.

The following is a list of remedies that should definitely not be taken during pregnancy. There are some here that are not mentioned elsewhere in this book: I have included them to make the list as comprehensive as possible. The list continues over the page.

aloes, Barbados or Cape	blue cohosh	euonymous bark
arbor vitae	broom	feverfew
autumn crocus	buchu	frangula bark
barberry	calumba root	fumitory
bearberry	cascara	ginseng
black cohosh	celery seeds	golden seal
bladderwrack	cinchona	greater celandine
blood root	cotton root	holy thistle
	elecampane	jamaica dogwood

juniper	nutmeg	rosemary
life root	parsley	rue
liquorice	passion flower	sage
lobelia	pennyroyal	senna, leaf or pods
male fern	poke root	southernwood
marjoram	prickly ash bark	tansy
meadow saffron	pulsatilla	thuja
mistletoe	quassia	thyme
motherwort	raspberry leaves	wormwood
(in the first eight months)	*(in the first eight months)*	
mugwort	rhubarb root	

The list may seem long, but it is only a small number compared to the enormous amount of herbal remedies that are quite safe to use. There are plenty of safe remedies capable of achieving just as effective results as any on this list.

Herbal teas make pleasant drinks as an alternative to ordinary tea and coffee, which some women find quite unpalatable during pregnancy. Try the fruit-flavoured or spicy ones if you like a strong flavour, or chicory if you want a similar taste to coffee.

Numerous herbal remedies are ideally suited to helping with the problems of pregnancy. Most women will experience one or two of the minor problems: this is because the physiological changes a woman's body goes through in the time leading up to the birth are enormous. Usually it is a matter of a degree of discomfort rather than dangerous problems. Antenatal services are intended to detect and treat anything that is potentially serious. Some of the commoner problems are considered here and some can be found in Chapter 7 if they are not exclusively problems of pregnancy.

BLOOD PRESSURE PROBLEMS

Your blood pressure will be checked regularly throughout the pregnancy, during routine visits to an antenatal clinic. Usually in the first months it will be lower than normal and if the normal for you is low to start with (as it is in many quite healthy people) this may trigger feelings of faintness. These are particularly noticeable if you have been bending over and then stand up too suddenly, or when you get up out of a hot bath. To avoid faintness, make sure you change position slowly and hold on to something to steady yourself if possible. Avoid very hot baths and hot stuffy atmospheres generally. Don't let yourself go for too long without having something to eat, because if you have low blood pressure the feeling of faintness can be triggered by a low blood sugar level. The warming spicy-tasting herbal remedies will help against faintness. Regular doses of ginger as a tea or as crystallized ginger are helpful. The combination of remedies known as Composition Essence (obtainable from herb/health shops) taken in a tepid drink is also recommended.

High blood pressure is a cause of greater concern: it must be checked regularly. Try to get as much rest and relaxation as possible (not easy if you have young children to look after, but use every chance you get). The safe and gentle herbal remedies that help to correct high blood pressure are limeflowers, cramp bark and yarrow. If stress is a possible cause of the problem try valerian as well.

CONSTIPATION

The approach taken in pregnancy should be more cautious than you would normally be. The stimulating laxatives are to be avoided, as any substance that has a stimulating action on the muscles of the bowel could have a similar effect on the womb. This applies equally to herbal or nonherbal laxatives. Thus senna and cascara should not be taken. Make sure you are having enough to drink - a total of about 2.25 litres/4 pints of fluid a day is advised. Try increasing your intake of fruit and vegetables to start with, particularly items like rhubarb, prunes and figs. This will add to the fibre you are eating.

If more than this is needed, take more fibre in the form of psyllium seeds rather than bran. Psyllium seeds form a soft gel which helps keep the stool moving through easily and is much less harsh to the lining of the digestive tract than bran.

If these steps don't solve the problem, try taking a liver tonic remedy like dandelion root or yellow dock root. These are less irritating than laxatives but still effective.

FLUID RETENTION

This is sometimes an aspect of blood pressure problems (see entry above), but even women with normal pressure tend to get some degree of swelling in the ankles towards the end of the pregnancy. The best remedy is dandelion leaves. The amount required to get the benefit varies from person to person, so take a cupful every three hours until you notice that you are passing more water and that the swelling is subsiding. You might need a smaller maintenance dose periodically - take a cupful as required.

INDIGESTION

Flatulence and heartburn can occur throughout pregnancy. The effects of the hormone changes may be responsible and in later stages the size and weight of the growing baby put pressure on the stomach and intestines. With this in mind, avoid lifting heavy objects or bending over - these put more pressure on the abdomen. Cut out rich, fatty and sugary foods: keep to a fairly plain diet to avoid unnecessary demands on the digestive system. Avoid ordinary tea and coffee, which can have very irritating effects on the digestion. Make your meals small and frequent – this avoids the overloading of the stomach that can otherwise be a cause of disturbances. Try any of the drinks indicated for morning sickness in the entry below, with the exception of large quantities of ginger: this could be too 'hot' and irritating if you are having problems with acidity. In addition try meadowsweet tea – this is the prime remedy for acidity and heartburn.

MORNING SICKNESS

This can start early in the pregnancy. Women vary enormously in their susceptibility to this problem and there is a wide range of remedies that have proved helpful in treating it. The first piece of advice is to have something plain to eat (like a cracker or oatcake) before you get out of bed in the morning. Then try herbal teas such as chamomile, caraway or coriander. Bitter drinks like *gentian can be useful while spices like ginger – either a few slices of the fresh root added to a drink or a piece of crystallized ginger to chew on – are well worth trying. Slippery elm powder is very soothing to the stomach and helps to reduce the tenderness that is felt after vomiting.

You may need to try several of these remedies until you find one that is palatable and effective. Women's tastes are so variable in early pregnancy that what appeals to one can be quite unpleasant to another.

CAUTION

Gentian is not suitable if you have a gastric or duodenal ulcer.

STRETCH MARKS

These occur when pressure on the skin becomes greater than its elasticity can cope with. The strength of the skin is due to protein fibres called collagen. To form collagen, Vitamin C and a related substance called rutin are required. These are both found in fruits, especially the citrus family, so make sure your diet contains plenty of them. In addition, use an oil on your breasts and abdomen that contains comfrey and Vitamin E. These will help to keep the skin supple and healthy, cutting down on the risk of permanent marks.

PREPARING FOR THE BIRTH

Until recent times it was traditional for women to take *raspberry leaf tea for the last month of their pregnancy. This remedy was widely known to help ease the process of birth – indeed, it was the last remaining bit of knowledge about herbs in my own family. There are other remedies that can be combined with it to help even more. This combination will help to make the muscles of the womb do their work with maximum efficiency and may reduce the pain experienced. It should be taken two or three times a day throughout the *last month of pregnancy, but not before. Mix 25g (1oz) each of *motherwort, black haw and raspberry leaves. Add half a teaspoon of powdered ginger to this, or add two slices of fresh root ginger to each cup of tea made from the mixture.

CAUTION

Do not take raspberry leaf or motherwort any earlier than the last month of pregnancy.

Four out of five births are free of problems and the option of having as natural a birth as possible can be fulfilled. If you turn out to be one of the women who have a difficult labour or birth and need medical interventions as a result, don't feel that you have failed somehow. Nobody can predict beforehand exactly how things will go. However well you look after yourself and even if you plan for a natural birth, bear in mind that if problems do occur it may be necessary to accept that your plans might have

to be changed if medical interventions are required.
In the end the criterion of success is that mother and
baby should both be well, however that end is reached.

AFTER THE BIRTH

Raspberry leaf and motherwort tea can be
continued right through the time after the birth, as
they will both help the womb return to normal.

It is also generally beneficial to add some healing
herbs to the water in which you bathe. This will
help the perineal area, between the vagina and the
back passage, recover from the enormous
stretching it has been through. It will also speed up
the healing of any cuts that might have been made
here. Make a double strength tea of comfrey and
marigold and add this to the bathwater.

HERBS FOR CHILDHOOD ILLNESSES

The range of remedies I recommend for children's problems is much
narrower than those that can be taken by adults. I don't like to use anything
that has a very strong action and I keep to those that have an acceptable
taste: however much a herb might help is irrelevant if you can't persuade a
child to take a second dose.

CAUTION

*If you are not completely sure about the causes of a child's illness,
consult a doctor or herbal practitioner.*

There are two remedies that are useful in a wide range of childhood
problems: chamomile and limeflowers. Try them in combination with any
others suggested as your first line of treatment. They both have a calming

and soothing effect that is invaluable, as children tend to get very miserable or distressed when they feel ill. Their gentle relaxing action is also helpful when children are overtired. For babies you can make a quarter-strength tea, strain it carefully and give it on a teaspoon or add it to a bottle formula instead of plain water. Alternatively, make a normal strength tea and add it to the baby's bathwater – he or she will breathe in the vapours and absorb the remedies through the skin. From toddler age onwards children can be given half-strength herbal teas as well as other drinks, so that they get used to a number of different tastes (assuming they are prepared to cooperate!).

The following list will cover most of the common illnesses of childhood. Bear in mind that it is not intended to give you information about diagnosing illnesses – it is not an alternative to seeking professional medical attention for your child.

CHICKENPOX

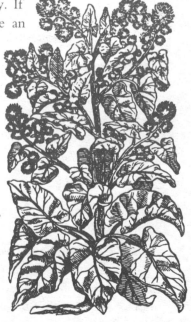

The degree to which children feel ill when they have this infectious disease varies enormously. If the child has a fever there will probably be an accompanying headache and lack of appetite. Try limeflowers or catmint to help keep the fever within safe limits, in which case the other symptoms should not get too severe. Give plenty of drinks – diluted fruit juices as well as the herbal teas. Keeping up a good fluid intake is much more important than eating solid food at this time.

The number of fluid-filled spots varies tremendously as well. These can be very itchy, but should not be scratched as this may result in scarring. Swab them liberally with distilled witch-hazel (or the gel form), or try chickweed ointment. A tepid bath in water containing bicarbonate of soda often helps to reduce the itching.

COLDS

For children over the age of eight years, try a few drops of Composition Essence (obtainable from herb/health shops) in a drink of hot fruit juice as the first step. For younger children, try a more gentle remedy – cinnamon has a similar but milder action. Use garlic as an anti-infective remedy: give about a quarter of a clove a day to children aged four years, half a clove to children aged ten years and adult doses over the age of fourteen. The garlic can be crushed and added to a little honey to make it more palatable. For children under the age of four years and for those who really hate the taste, the garlic can be applied externally rather than eaten. Crush the clove and add it to a small amount of olive oil. This can then be massaged into the front and back of the chest.

For children who seem to have a low resistance to this type of infection, try the following supplements taken regularly for several months: garlic, Vitamins A and C (ideally taken as plenty of fresh fruit and vegetables in the diet, but as a supplement of about 200-400mg Vitamin C and 1,000 i.u. Vitamin A daily if this is not achieved) and multiminerals containing zinc in particular.

COLIC

Some babies can be particularly prone to this problem. The traditional formula of gripe-water contains dill and a little ginger, both of which are excellent carminatives. Dill, caraway or chamomile can also be given in the form of herbal teas (made to one quarter of the usual strength to start with) which, if strained carefully, can be added to a baby's bottle formula or given on a teaspoon. Don't use ginger – it is too 'hot' in any but the tiniest amounts.

CAUTION

If the discomfort is accompanied by vomiting and you suspect an infection seek professional attention for the baby.

If the cause is not an infection (for which you must seek professional help) there is a possibility that it may be an intolerance to a particular food. Cows' milk allergy can cause colic, so if the baby is having a formula milk try changing to one based on soya - there are several brands available. If the baby is breast-fed there is a chance that the cause of the problem might be in the mother's diet. In any case, the mother should drink plenty of the carminative herbal teas like caraway, fennel and coriander, as some of the constituents will be passed on to the baby through the milk.

CONSTIPATION

This problem in children should be treated first through the diet. Give plenty of fruit, including items like prunes, figs, dates and rhubarb (including the juice). Choose wholegrain breakfast cereals rather than the cornflakes type and try wholegrain or granary bread. If this doesn't solve the problem, use psyllium seeds, which can be given in a drink to which fruit juice has been added to make it more palatable (the seeds don't have any taste, but they can look rather off-putting).

CAUTION

If the constipation needs treatment for longer than a week or is causing a lot of distress to the child, seek help from your doctor or herbal practitioner.

COUGHS

The two remedies most suitable for children are aniseed and *coltsfoot. Both will help to loosen tight phlegm and soothe the dry, tickly cough that often prevents children (and parents) from getting a good night's sleep. Liquorice is another remedy that has a beneficial action on the lungs. Buy pure liquorice sticks from a herb/health shop - the liquorice you buy from the sweet shop hasn't got enough real liquorice in it to produce the benefit. Give it only in small quantities to start with - it sometimes has a slight laxative effect.

CAUTION

Long-term use of coltsfoot is not advised.

CRADLE CAP

Sometimes a baby's scalp gets very dry and flaky, or it may become inflamed. There are several applications to try on the scalp to relieve this. Pure Vitamin E oil is an excellent gentle moisturizer and protector for the skin. Marigold and chamomile creams help to calm irritation and inflammation. Witch-hazel (probably easier to use in the gel form) is a good astringent to help reduce inflammation and give some protection to the surface of the skin if it has been irritated by any particular soaps, lanolin, or wool, etc.

CUTS AND GRAZES

The best remedy to use when cleaning a dirty wound is tincture of myrrh, but be warned that it will cause a few moments' stinging. If there is a red, swollen area of inflammation around the wound apply some chickweed ointment to reduce it. The healing of the wound can be encouraged by applying comfrey ointment.

DIGESTIVE PROBLEMS

Most children complain of tummy aches or feeling sick occasionally, and for some it is a persistent frequent problem. There may be stress problems, infections or food intolerances involved, so if this happens frequently, give consideration to whether or not specific recurring circumstances seem to trigger it. If particular foods seem to be causing the problem, they must be removed from the diet. If this results in a big change in the diet, I would suggest a consultation with a professional dietician to check that the new diet is well balanced and nourishing enough for the needs of the child.

The first line of treatment, which should bring some relief whatever the cause of the problem, is chamomile and cinnamon tea, interspersed with slippery elm powder drinks (taken as a separate drink or mixed with yogurt and honey, according to the preference of the child). These both have an excellent soothing effect and can be taken repeatedly without fear of side-effects.

Sometimes using the relaxing remedies - try limeflowers and lemon balm - is a useful step.

C A U T I O N

If the symptoms remain severe an infection could be present and professional attention should be considered.

E A R A C H E

This is the most unpleasant of all the symptoms associated with upper respiratory infections. Because of the risk of damage to the delicate mechanism of hearing and balance in the ears, in my opinion it always requires professional attention. In addition to this, the best herbal treatment is to massage a warmed mixture of garlic and a little olive oil onto the bony area behind the ear. This will be absorbed through the skin and help clear any infection in that area. If a child is prone to recurrent earaches a regular internal dose of garlic - about half a raw clove a day, or one tablet or capsule at night - will help reduce this tendency.

CAUTION

Always seek professional advice if a child has earache.

FEVERS

Some children have a very ready tendency to develop a fever as part of their generalized reaction to infectious disease. A moderately high temperature helps to create an environment within the body that is hostile to the infectious organism, so it is part of the body's defence mechanism. But if the temperature gets too high it poses a risk to the child, so remedies to regulate it are important. There are several that are pleasant-tasting and effective. Try limeflowers, catmint and elderflowers, taken every three hours. these should stabilize the temperature, even if it stays a little higher than normal. They can all be sweetened with honey or fruit juice. In addition, try sponging the child with tepid water if required.

CAUTION

Always seek professional assistance if a child has a very high fever.

NAPPY RASH

The degree to which babies suffer from this varies tremendously, but there aren't many who escape it completely. It often seems to coincide with teething. Make sure that the nappy area is washed free of urine every time the nappy is changed. Rinse the area with plain warm water after using the cleanser, and use a very gentle one to rule out the possibility that this is adding to the skin reaction. Apply one of the soothing herbal creams - chamomile, marigold and St John's wort are all good. You may need to apply something over the top of this to act like a barrier cream - wheatgerm oil, which is very rich in Vitamin E, is worth trying.

RASHES

These temporary skin problems can come and go quite mysteriously, but can cause a good deal of itching and irritation in children who are prone to them. As with many skin problems, there may be several possible causes and any observations you can make about these will be helpful in the future. Some children react badly to particular fibres against their skin: wool and artificial fibres provoke most of the reactions and cotton is usually the best tolerated. Particular types of soaps, bubble-baths, washing powders, etc. can cause irritation, so if a rash develops think about whether or not any of these have been changed recently. New foods might be responsible, and any of these problems can be aggravated by stress and worries that the child is subject to. Sometimes the reaction can result from a pleasant type of overexcitement, like having a birthday party or other special treat - in which case the rash generally calms down by itself in due course.

Whatever the cause, the severity of the rash can usually be reduced by using one of the soothing herbal ointments. If it is very itchy, try first swabbing it with witch-hazel and then apply chickweed ointment. If you have inflamed and 'burning' skin, use chamomile. If it looks very dry, try pure Vitamin E oil. Marigold and St John's wort are both valuable skin healing remedies too.

SORE THROATS

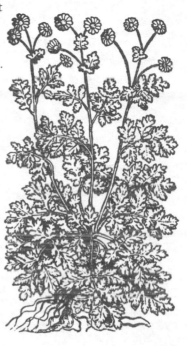

For sore throats, follow the suggestions given under the entry for Colds above, except for using Composition Essence (the effect of this can be too irritating on an already inflamed throat). In addition, use raspberry leaf tea as an astringent remedy to soothe the inflammation in the throat. Tincture of myrrh can be used as a gargle for children over the age of seven - make it very dilute, about one quarter of a teaspoon of the tincture to one tablespoon of water and is also useful to soothe the inflammation and fight off the infection. In addition, various herbal pastilles can be bought in a herb/health shop. Most of these will bring relief to the immediate symptoms and help to improve the condition of the membranes lining the throat.

The supplements recommended under Colds are worth taking long term if sore throats are a recurrent problem.

TEETHING

The discomfort experienced in the gums can make a toddler very distressed. Try chamomile or limeflowers as calming remedies. Chamomile can also have a soothing anti-inflammatory effect on the gums. Sometimes catarrhal symptoms can accompany the teething - elderflowers may help this.

A Herbal
First Aid Kit

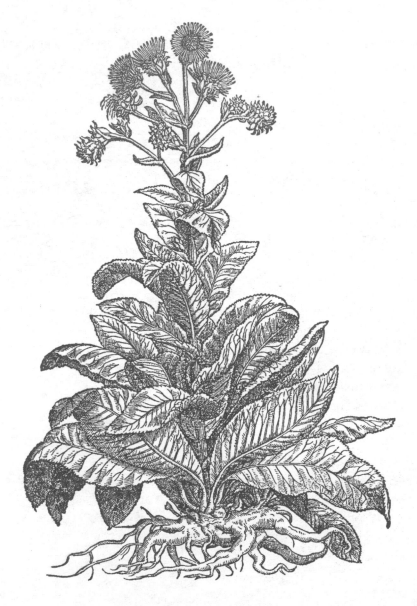

The well-stocked first aid kit should of course contain all the usual equipment for dealing with minor injuries: first aid manuals produced by the Red Cross or St John's give details. In addition to herbal remedies that are helpful to use on minor injuries I have included some that are valuable in the treatment of infections. These are worth having to hand to take at the first sign of the onset of an infection: used this way they can best ease the course of the illness. Herbal items that are useful are suggested as follows (also see under the alphabetical entries in Chapters 6 and 7).

CAUTION

In an emergency there are no medicines that can replace the invaluable skills learnt on first aid training courses. My advice is therefore to contact your local branch of the Red Cross or St John's Ambulance Brigade and join one of their courses. The information about herbal remedies given here will fit well alongside the use of first aid skills for the less severe problems you may frequently have to deal with in your home.

ARNICA OINTMENT

This is invaluable for speeding up the healing of bruises and therefore very useful for people involved in sports where such injuries are likely. The injured area should be treated with a cold pack or held under cold water until the immediate pain has subsided, then arnica can be applied as long as the skin overlying the affected area has not been broken.

CAUTION

Do not use arnica on broken skin.

BITTER TONICS

I have given this name rather than that of an individual bitter remedy as there are several that have a similar benefit. These herbs are useful for a hangover. Symptoms of overindulgence can be headaches, nausea or vomiting, and are due either to dehydration or to the irritating effect of alcohol on the digestive system and liver. Bitter remedies work by stimulating the liver to speed up the breakdown of alcohol. As such they are most effective when taken in advance of the alcohol - hence the European custom of taking very bitter-tasting drinks at the beginning of the evening. They will help the next day too, though.

Bitters are also useful to counteract feverish conditions and as an aid to convalescence after a debilitating illness. The standard bitter remedy is *gentian root, though dandelion root or *hops are also recommended.

CAUTION

Do not take gentian if you have a gastric or duodenal ulcer.
Hops should not be taken by people who are prone to depression.

BONESET HERB

This is the most useful remedy to bring down a high temperature. Take it at the first sign of the onset of fever in cases of head-colds, sore throats, chest infections, etc. It is also useful in helping to reduce catarrhal problems associated with respiratory infections.

Chamomile Herb

Although probably more thought of as an alternative to tea, chamomile is useful for a range of minor internal and external problems. It is well worth having available at short notice as it is one of the most widely applicable remedies for all types of digestive problems. Take it as a tea for problems of nausea, indigestion or colic, or for digestive infections involving diarrhoea and vomiting. It can also help reduce headaches and problems of nervous tension or anxiety. If a strong tea is made this can be used as a lotion on the skin, and is worth trying for any type of skin irritation like nettle rash or contact dermatitis. A cream containing extracts of chamomile is also available from health and chemist shops for this purpose.

Chickweed Ointment

This has proved invaluable for some cases of skin irritation. It is the remedy which has the highest reputation to help ease itching and can be used for nettle rash or contact dermatitis, and on itchy grazes and minor wounds. It has helped reduce reactions to insect bites for some people.

Comfrey Ointment

Of all the herbal ointments, this is the most useful for stimulating the repair processes in damaged skin, muscles and ligaments. Problems such as cuts and grazes, torn muscles or ligaments will benefit by healing more quickly. Even in non-specific muscular aches and pains it is worth trying comfrey. It should be applied regularly, twice a day, until the affected area feels normal again. It is very useful for sports people who risk frequent injury but cannot be out of action for too long. It is reputed to reduce the risk of scar-formation if used regularly on the injured area. Keep up its use until the problem is completely resolved to get the maximum benefit.

Composition Essence

Although now comparatively obscure, this mixture was well known in the past as a remedy to use against the harmful effects of exposure to cold. People vary in their susceptibility to the effects of cold, but the epidemics of respiratory illnesses and the worsening of many problems like arthritis that occur in the winter show that for some, a measure of protection is very helpful.

The mixture, which can be obtained from herb/health shops, has a spicy flavour and only small quantities should be taken at a time. Try adding about a quarter of a teaspoonful to a drink of hot fruit juice - the combination of flavours is delicious. This should be taken at the first sign of the onset of head-colds, chest infections, etc. Repeat the dose every three hours for the first day.

The other situation in which the mixture helps is when you have been out in cold or damp weather and feel very chilled - this type of 'cold' does not involve an infection; the reaction is simply due to the reduction in temperature. Take a drink of composition essence as soon as you can and then every three hours until you have recovered. People who are susceptible to chilblains will benefit from taking this treatment three times a day regularly throughout the winter.

FRIARS' BALSAM

This is easily obtainable from any chemist shop. It is used in the form of a *steam inhalation, to help with respiratory problems. Details of how to prepare this are in the entry for Benzoin in Chapter 6. Use friars' balsam to help reduce discomfort and congestion in cases of catarrh, sinusitis, head-colds and chesty coughs. It soothes irritated membranes and loosens mucus, resulting in easier breathing.

CAUTION

Some people with asthma may find that steam is irritating to their chests. Steam inhalations should not be used in these cases.

Used at the first sign of the onset of an infection, it may help to reduce the overall severity of the problem. It can also be used similarly to tincture of myrrh as an external antiseptic lotion.

Garlic

Many people take garlic capsules or tablets routinely for its beneficial action on the circulation. The properties I recommend it for here concern its ability to help fight off infections. Take it at the first sign of the onset of head-colds, sore throats, chest infections, etc. Two or three high-strength tablets are generally sufficient to get the benefit. Alternatively you can take one or two whole raw cloves a day, divided into several doses. It is also very helpful in cases of digestive system infections – the tablets are probably more palatable than the raw cloves in this situation.

Marigold Ointment

This healing ointment is particularly useful against fungal infections of the skin, like athlete's foot. It also helps the skin recover after minor burns or other injuries. It is worth trying on irritating rashes and eczema as well. If varicose veins in the legs are injured, marigold is the best remedy to apply regularly, though professional attention may also be required.

Myrrh (Tincture of)

A small bottle of this is invaluable in all households, as it is the most useful antiseptic and healing herbal remedy. It can still be purchased at many chemist shops, as it is a recognized pharmaceutical preparation. It can be taken internally in very small amounts to help fight infection, but its main use is for external application. If minor wounds and grazes need cleaning or bathing, add about half a teaspoonful of tincture of myrrh to the water you use. It can be used similarly on spots, acne, insect bites and abscesses to remove bacteria from the surface of the skin. Apply it to mouth ulcers – use it neat to get the best results, though you may have to put up with a minute or two of stinging. Otherwise dilute it to the same strength as for the skin application and use it as a mouthwash. It will help against all mouth and gum infections this way. Use it also as a gargle in the event of a sore throat.

SLIPPERY ELM POWDER

This remedy is the most universally applicable one for digestive problems, short of acute emergencies. In all cases of minor disturbances such as the results of overindulgence, excess acidity and indigestion, vomiting, etc., slippery elm should be taken. It will help calm the unpleasant symptoms of a digestive infection, though as it is not an anti-infective remedy it will not get rid of the infection. It will bring about a feeling of comfort in the stomach, and calm the severity of diarrhoea without preventing the body from ridding itself of the harmful micro-organisms (which is what the diarrhoea reaction achieves). It is very well tolerated by children, but if they don't like it in the form of a drink try mixing it with some plain live yogurt and a little honey. This is an excellent nutritious combination, very soothing in most cases of digestive disturbance, and it tastes delicious.

WITCH-HAZEL

Of all the herbal preparations available, this must be the best known. It is available from all chemist shops as the traditional liquid distilled witch-hazel. There is also now a very useful gel form on sale. The soothing anti-inflammatory action of witch-hazel makes it useful in a number of situations. Any minor injury where there is pain and swelling, such as sprains, muscle strains and bruises, will be eased by soaking in cold water initially, then applying witch-hazel liberally. It will help staunch the flow of blood from minor wounds, though standard first aid advice nowadays is not to use any applications on wounds. It is the most soothing application to areas of sunburn: cover the affected area with a piece of lint or other suitable cloth and keep it moistened with witch-hazel - you can pour on more as the cloth dries out. It is also useful in any type of skin irritation and can be applied to the itchy swellings that sometimes develop after insect bites.

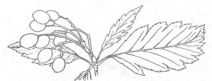

HERBS AND SKIN CARE

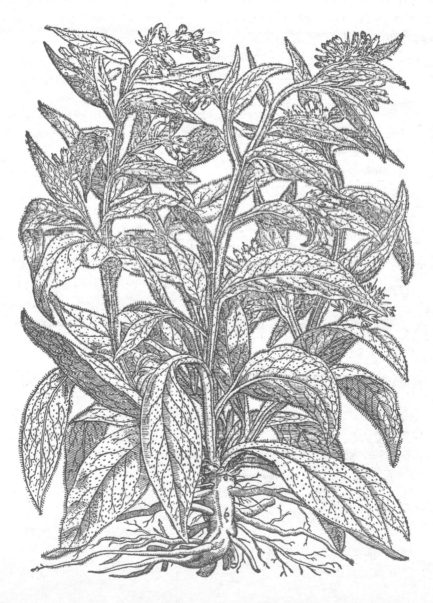

In the past many of the cosmetics and toiletries used on the skin were derived from herbs. For instance, the botanical name for the deadly nightshade is *Belladonna* - meaning 'beautiful lady' - a reference to the use of eyedrops made from the plant to dilate the pupils and make the eyes look very dark. The contrast between dark eyes and a very pale skin (achieved by applying ointments made with a base of white lead) was considered a mark of beauty. Unfortunately for the beautiful lady, both preparations were harmful and she paid a high price for her appearance in terms of her health.

Recipes for home-made preparations, very similar to some I have included in this book, were published in the 'do-it-yourself' books of previous centuries. Nowadays we are lucky that if we make our own it is through choice - we have the option of buying ready-made items, whereas our predecessors had to make their own or go without. Luckily for them, there were numerous easily available herbs that can benefit the skin. These were usually remedies having either an astringent or an anti-inflammatory action, or those that moisturized and protected the skin. They were prepared as teas to use as lotions, or as infused oils or ointments. If they were to be kept for some time they needed to include some preservative substance to prevent the growth of micro-organisms. Many preparations contain a small amount of alcohol for this purpose, such as the elderflower water recipe given in the relevant entry in Chapter 6.

Basic treatments for correcting skin problems are given in this chapter. Remember the importance of general health points, such as a good diet with plenty of fresh fruit and vegetables and the right amount of exercise. The skin is one of the most extensive organs of the body and is greatly affected by what you eat and do. Stress problems can also have a great influence on the skin. The causes of diseases such as eczema, psoriasis and transitory rashes are still largely unknown, and it may take a fair amount of detective work to pin down what specific influences are affecting the skin of a particular individual.

DRY SKIN

This type of skin is most commonly associated with eczema (which simply means inflammation of the skin). When the normal oils are not produced, the skin is much more vulnerable to damage from influences like cold winds, contact with chemicals, etc. If you have dry skin that occasionally develops into eczema, it is worth taking notice of the circumstances in which the flare-up occurs. it may be particular foods, chemicals or types of stress that provoke it. To keep your skin as well protected as possible, try a moisturizing cream that contains Vitamin E oil (for eczema I recommend trying pure Vitamin E oil on the affected area). The North American herbalists used to recommend a tea made of sunflower seeds and burdock seeds as a drink to improve oil production in the skin. Sunflower seeds certainly make a nourishing snack, as they are rich in Vitamin E and a range of valuable minerals.

OILY SKIN

You need an astringent remedy to apply to oily skin - this will remove any oil accumulated on the surface, keep the skin clean and tighten the surface. In the long term this can help reduce the amount of secretions produced by the oil glands. Try witch-hazel, or a cosmetic preparation based on it (this is one of the most gentle yet effective of all the herbal astringents). Oily skin tends to develop blackheads, where the oil in a pore reacts with air to produce a black colour on its surface. These will be less noticeable if the pores are tight rather than lax and again astringents will help.

The gel form of witch-hazel can be used as a face-pack. Another traditionally used material for a pack is finely ground oatmeal. Mix this with water and a little bit of slippery elm powder (which helps soothe inflamed skin and will give a more workable consistency), apply to the skin and leave for about fifteen minutes. Gently wash it off with cool water and pat the skin dry. Elderflower water (a recipe for this is given under Elder in Chapter 6) is another traditional astringent used on the skin, to help reduce blemishes as well as counteract oiliness. The two can easily be combined.

Sometimes if the skin is excessively oily the problem can be alleviated by taking herbal remedies internally. The most suitable are those that used to be known as the 'blood purifiers'. Various combinations are still available over the counter, in the form of tablets or dried herbs to take as teas. These are well worth trying if you have a persistent or severe problem.

PUFFY SKIN

People suffering from allergies sometimes get swollen skin, particularly around the eyelids. The same reaction can cause the eyes themselves to be itchy and bloodshot. The first treatment for this is to spread a cloth soaked in cold water over the face. It doesn't cure the problem but it brings an immediate sense of relief by reducing the irritation. Then try applying a cloth or pad of suitable material soaked in distilled witch-hazel. Follow this with some chamomile cream or ointment around the eyes. Some people have found that the 'cleansing' remedies like clivers, burdock, yellow dock and red clover are helpful in alleviating allergic skin problems.

The other cause of puffy skin on the face is a type of *fluid retention. This can be relieved by taking dandelion leaf tea, but you should consult your doctor if you think this is your problem.

CAUTION

Seek professional advice if you suspect fluid retention.

RED NOSE

This is usually due to the dilation of blood vessels in the local area. It happens mainly in the winter as a result of exposure to the cold weather.

The most successful treatment I have found is a combination of herbal remedies and vitamin supplements. Take Vitamin C in a moderate dose – about 500mg daily – and also take about 100mg of rutin a day. These two substances are involved in the formation of the protein fibres that give structural strength to the skin and blood vessels. Try yarrow and a little ginger as a tea to regulate the dilation of the blood vessels.

There are other conditions that cause a reddening of the skin because of inflammation. These are more akin to eczema and generally respond to the same range of remedies (see Dry Skin above).

SENSITIVE SKIN

Some people have to be very careful about what they apply to their skin, because of the risk of resulting inflammation. Recently, cosmetics companies have become more aware of these problems and numerous products for sensitive skins are now available. These are specifically formulated to avoid ingredients like lanolin (oil obtained from sheep's wool) and other animal products that can cause sensitivity reactions. With some people the skin reaction is due to a classic allergy and may be one of a range of symptoms. With others it is more akin to an inability to cope with the irritation caused by certain substances. The skin usually looks red and inflamed and it can feel itchy, hot or stinging to the sufferer. It can be swollen, blotchy, dry or weeping in severe cases. If it is badly affected, you may need to seek help from a medical practitioner to prevent further problems developing. Otherwise, try swabbing the affected area with witch-hazel to calm the inflammation and help protect the skin. Then apply either chamomile or marigold lotions, made in the same way as a double-strength tea. These are both very soothing and healing to inflamed skin and can be used regularly if they prove beneficial. Both are also available in ointment form, suitable for dry skin. If the skin has the appearance of urticaria (nettle-rash), try a tea made of nettles, both taken internally and applied as a lotion – this has been helpful to several of my patients.

SLOW-TO-HEAL SKIN

Dietary factors and general health can influence this problem. If your skin seems to bruise very easily, try increasing your intake of fruit and salad vegetables, which will automatically increase your Vitamin C intake. If you have citrus fruits, apricots, grapes, tomatoes and broccoli regularly you will also be getting plenty of the bioflavonoids that work with Vitamin C to form the strength-giving fibres in the walls of the blood vessels. The outcome should be a reduced tendency to bruising of the skin.

Poor circulation can be the cause of impaired skin healing, particularly on the lower legs. This is a well-known consequence if the ankles are swollen with fluid for long periods of time. The circulation of blood and tissue fluid in the lower legs slows down, so that the skin is poorly nourished and very delicate. If it is then injured, the healing processes are impaired because nutrients are not being delivered and waste products are accumulating. In this unfortunate situation the injury sometimes develops into an *ulcer. Professional medical attention is required, as the ulcer will at the least need special dressings, but herbal remedies can play a valuable role in treatment.

The first requirement for recovery is to clear the excess fluid from the ankles, by taking dandelion leaf tea and following the advice to this purpose given in other chapters. When the ankles are normal again, the blood supply will be much more efficient and able to support the healing processes. Keep the ulcer clean by bathing it with dilute tincture of myrrh – about half a teaspoonful to two tablespoons of warm water. Be warned that these ulcers can be very painful and that bathing them might sting somewhat. If the area is inflamed, try a poultice made of slippery elm powder mixed with double-strength chamomile tea. Apply this to the ulcer and wash it off with warm water after ten or fifteen minutes. Then use comfrey ointment to promote skin healing before covering the area with a dressing. If this routine is followed regularly you have the best chance of seeing an improvement.

C A U T I O N

Seek professional advice if you develop an ulcer on your skin.

SPOTS

If these occur as a result of oily skin, follow the advice for that condition given above. Otherwise, try to observe what may be connected with the onset of the spots when they flare up, noting any changes in diet, routine, stress problems, etc. A woman should also check whether the outbreak is connected with her monthly hormone cycle. If a cause can be located and thereafter avoided, the chances of improving the skin condition are greatly increased.

Use witch-hazel on the surface of the spots: this calms the inflammation and can reduce the tenderness. If the spots have infected heads, bathe them with dilute tincture of myrrh - half a teaspoonful to a tablespoon of water.

The spots may be an indication of the need for some internal treatment. As with oily skin, a course of 'blood-purifying' herbs may be beneficial to correct the problem. This group of remedies, including burdock, clivers, nettles and yellow dock, helps to improve the metabolism and elimination of waste products through the excretory organs of the body.

CONSULTING A HERBAL PRACTITIONER

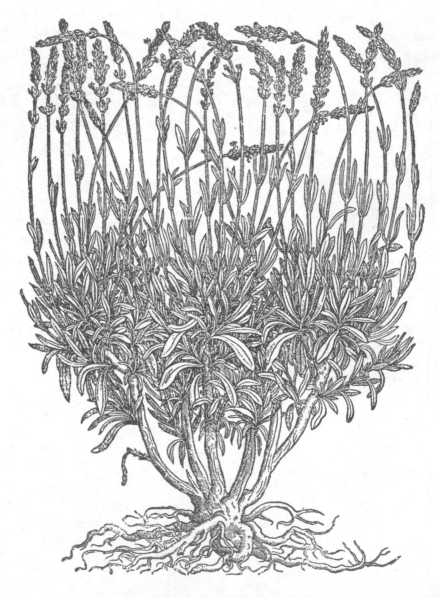

The remedies and illnesses mentioned in this book cover only a limited range of the problems that herbs can help with. By all means try the suggestions here first, but if your problem is complex or long-standing you may need to visit a professional herbalist to get the most effective treatment. This chapter gives you some information about what this will entail.

Firstly, you need to locate a qualified practitioner. Of all the different types of complementary medicine available, herbal medicine seems to have the lowest profile. Most people think of it only in terms of what is available in the herb/health shop, without realizing that there are highly trained practitioners available for consultation. There are about 500 herbal practitioners in the UK, with more qualifying each year. This sounds a small number, but compared to the much smaller number practising twenty years ago it represents an enormous increase!

It is rare to see any sort of advertising by herbalists, so you will have to know where to look to get the required information. Your local Yellow Pages will have an entry for Herbalists, and this is the easiest way to locate one. Look for the letters that come after the person's name: this will indicate what training and qualifications they have received. FNIMH or MNIMH stands for Fellow or Member of the National Institute of Medical Herbalists. MRCH stands for Member of the Register of Consultant Herbalists. The addresses of these organizations are given at the end of this book. If other qualifications are shown, you are free to ask about them when you contact the practitioner – everyone has the right to know about the professional background of the person to whom they are entrusting their health.

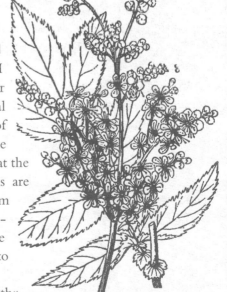

If you can't find anyone through the

Yellow Pages it may be that there are no practitioners in your immediate area and you will have to look further afield. If you write to the professional organizations enclosing a stamped addressed envelope, they will send you a list of their members working throughout the UK.

Training in herbal medicine nowadays involves a three- or four-year course. The subjects covered include those studied by orthodox medical students, such as anatomy, physiology, pathology and diagnosis. The specific naturopathic and herbal approaches are covered in studies of herbal *Materia Medica* and the philosophy of herbal medicine. The need to treat each person as an individual and to consider the underlying causes of disease are stressed here. Later in the training, more specialized subjects of particular relevance to herbal treatment are covered, such as skin disease and gynaecological problems. Alongside the academic work there is a programme of clinical training to impart the skills of interviewing and examining patients. Written and practical examinations cover the academic and clinical aspects of the work, and students must pass both to become qualified. It will be obvious that to be successful the student of herbal medicine must feel very committed to the work.

The first time you visit a herbalist the consultation will probably take about forty-five minutes to an hour. As well as talking in depth about all aspects of the problems you are concerned about, there will be numerous questions about your general health and constitution. Information about points such as how your digestion functions, whether you sleep well and how severely you feel the cold in the winter is very important to build up a picture of your particular health and constitution, so that your specific problems can be seen in this context.

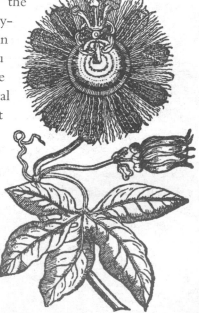

Most practitioners consider diet to be an important aspect of health, so this will be discussed and possibly some changes suggested. Similarly with exercise. There may be some examinations the practitioner needs to carry out – these will be similar to what a GP does, such as checking your blood pressure, listening to your heart, looking at a sore throat, etc. At the end of this, the herbalist should have a good idea of what the causes of your problem might be, and can therefore make a suitable combination of remedies to help put things right. The ability to identify the causes of the problem, and work out the best combination of remedies to treat them, is where the skill of the professional is required. The four years of training are all absolutely necessary to develop proficiency in such skills.

Most remedies used by practitioners in Britain are in the form of tinctures. These used to be a well-known form of preparation in orthodox medicine, but now only one or two survive in the contemporary *British Pharmacopoeia*. You may have come across the best-known one, tincture of myrrh, in other chapters of this book. Tinctures are prepared by soaking a specific amount of the herbal material in a specific amount of a liquid composed of water and pure alcohol. The usual quantities are 200g of the herb to 1 litre of liquid, though for a few remedies 100g to 1 litre is used.

The amount of alcohol in the liquid varies, depending on the type of constituents in the herb that are to be extracted into the liquid. If the required constituents are soluble in water the amount of alcohol is only 25 per cent, as the water will draw out the constituents of the herb quite adequately. In these preparations the alcohol is present largely to act as a preservative, so that the preparation will have a good shelf-life and there need be no concern about microbial contamination (the alcohol guarantees that the preparation is sterile). However, some constituents, such as resins, don't dissolve at all well in water, so a higher proportion of alcohol is necessary as a solvent. Some tinctures, including tincture of myrrh, must be 90 per cent alcohol to dissolve the resins. Thus for each plant used by herbalists, the amount of herb to liquid, and the amount of alcohol within that liquid are specified by the *British Herbal Pharmacopoeia*.

Generally, tinctures of different remedies combine together very well. Combining remedies is one of the key skills of the professional. I have given an idea of the types of remedies that go well together in Chapter 7 but there is far more to it than is covered there. For the professional herbalist, getting the combination right is a crucial matter. A prescription from a herbalist might contain six or more different remedies, as it will be designed to help with all the functional problems that the practitioner thinks are having an adverse influence on the disease in question. As an example, a typical combination for a stomach ulcer would include direct soothing remedies such as chamomile, marshmallow or slippery elm, plus something to counteract too much acidity, like meadowsweet. A promoter of healing – comfrey, for instance – and possibly some relaxing remedies such as passion flower will be included if it seems that stress is one of the causes.

The dosage of the combined tinctures suggested by most practitioners is usually a 5ml teaspoon three times a day. Although it may not taste pleasant, because it is a small amount most patients find it is fairly easy to take. I am interested to find that many people say they come to get used to the taste – if you have confidence that what you are taking is going to do you good, it is much easier to swallow.

The duration of the treatment is very variable: it depends on the nature of the illness. In self-limiting problems like coughs and colds no more than a week or two's medicine should be needed. For ailments such as recurrent infections it obviously takes longer to build up the normal resistance of the immune system. For long-term problems - eczema, arthritis, etc - it is hard to predict how long a person will need to take the medicine. My own guidelines are that for a long-term condition it can take up to three months to get the maximum benefit from the treatment, so although I see most patients on a monthly basis, it is at the three-month stage that the most crucial assessment is made (I'm glad to be able to say that most people find they get beneficial results from the treatment well before this time, though). If things are going well I might suggest a small reduction in the dosage of the medicine at this time, to see whether the improvement can be maintained. Further reductions can be made in due course, as the aim is to find the minimum dose that maintains a patient's health.

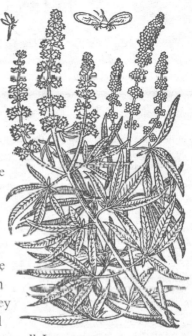

With the enormously varied range of problems that people bring to me, I find I have some patients who have been taking herbal medicine for years, and others who only need to come once or twice to solve their problems. Of course, there are some whom it doesn't seem able to help - I don't think there is any system of medicine that can be successful in all cases. I can't guarantee success, but what I set out to offer is the standard of attention and concern about my patients' problems. I give the undertaking to do all I can to help, using the remedies that I have been trained to prescribe. In the time I have been using them I have come to have great respect for and confidence in their powers to heal.

CHAPTER 12

CHINESE HERBAL MEDICINE

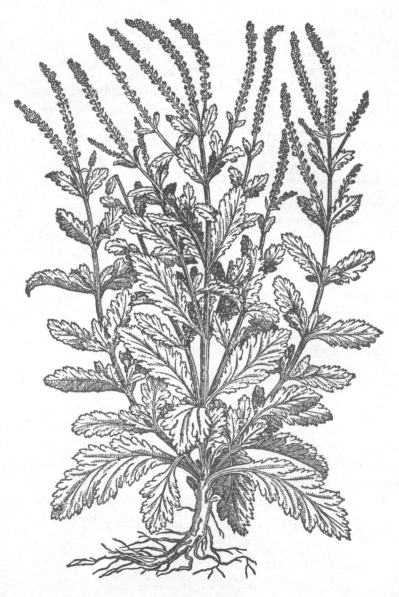

When I trained as a herbal practitioner about fifteen years ago, I learnt about one or two Chinese plants that happened to be well known and used by Western herbalists. We fitted them in with our Western approach and found them as helpful as any of our European herbs for their specific uses. Since then far more has been learnt about the wide range of medicinal plants used in China, and about the very different techniques of diagnosis and prescribing that are at the heart of the Chinese system.

This system has been developing over several millennia, accounts of the use of herbs in China date back more than 4,000 years. Like its Western counterpart it has been subject to a huge range of influences since that time, and traditional Chinese medicine has more aspects than just the acupuncture and herbs that we associate with it today. In the past trained, 'classical' medical thinkers were involved on the theoretical side; they did not actually see many patients. At the other extreme, as in the West, there were the local wise women who had no academic training but learnt about herbal remedies and acupuncture through apprenticeship, or from members of their families. There were spiritual healers too, and pilgrimages to sacred shrines were made in the hope of obtaining cures for illnesses, much as in the West. There were even street vendors selling cures among their wares.

In the 1930s and 40s when the Kuomintang regime of Chiang Kai Shek was in power, traditional medicine of all types was banned. It was considered old-fashioned and based on superstitions. When the Communists founded the People's Republic of China in 1949 it was reinstated. State patronage granted it a place alongside Western medicine in hospitals, and college training became available. Textbooks were written

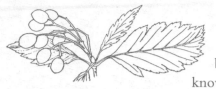

on the subject, which meant that some of the diversity was lost as Chinese medicine became more standardized. Nowadays the knowledge is open to all who choose to study it, whereas previously it was in the hands of practitioners who often preferred to keep their individual secrets and skills 'in the family'. Aspects of traditional medicine that have not harmonized well with this new approach have diminished. Under the new training system the concepts involved, although still very different from those in Western medicine, are narrower than the enormous range of ideas that was held in the past.

An earlier time of change occurred about 2,000 years ago during the Hang dynasty. It seems that the idea of the human body as a microcosm of or model for both the Chinese political order of the time and for the order of the universe was developed at about that time. Concepts of the 'order of the body' - that is, the interrelationships between the different organs - were part of this. The model had meaning that applied far beyond the scope of an individual's health. The idea of the correct balance between all parts of the body was central to the development of medical treatment, as it was also to the government of the country. The concept of the circulating 'qi' (see below) was developed and the technique of acupuncture soon followed. Herbal remedies, minerals and animal extracts were all used therapeutically within this model.

As the conceptual system is applied today, it still embodies a totally different view of health and disease to that of the West. In practice, the Chinese system is in basic agreement about the importance of points like diet and exercise as the foundations of good health. But the diagnostic processes of Chinese and Western herbal medicine often arrive at conclusions that are remarkably similar, though the techniques and concepts used are so different.

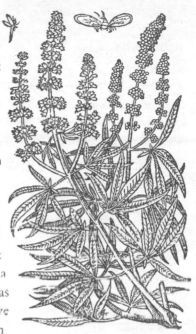

In modern-day China the two systems exist side by side. For instance, in Shanghai there are three universities teaching Western medicine and one teaching traditional Chinese medicine. All the students learning Western medicine spend six months of their training learning the basics of the traditional system. Most hospitals have a department where traditional medicine is practised and a pharmacy that supplies herbal as well as orthodox medicines. So city-dwellers still have access to traditional treatment, though Western treatment is probably the norm. In rural areas traditional medicine is still the main type of treatment, and here the medical practitioners may not have had an academic training. They are more likely to have learnt through apprenticeship, or to be continuing a family tradition of practice, probably in acupuncture and herbal medicine.

Among the general population herbal preparations are more readily thought of as a normal part of life than they are in the West. People use ginseng as a winter tonic, while in the summer herbal teas like peppermint are a popular drink. With the introduction of the Western way of life these customs may decline in the cities, but in the more traditional rural areas they will surely continue. Differences in food-preferences can already be seen, with city-dwellers in Shanghai reducing the amount of garlic in their food compared with rural areas. Ginger is used in cooking, but in Shanghai it is removed before the meal is served while in northern areas of China it is eaten with the rest of the food.

To understand traditional Chinese medicine it is necessary to know something of the Chinese thinking on how the universe functions. Although trying to pin these ideas down and give them fixed definitions is distorting them, I will attempt to give some information that might help.

In Chinese thought there are up to three aspects to everything that exists. The most material aspect is called jing: this is the substance of the bodies of living organisms, whether plants, animals or humans. Almost all of the work of Western medicine (by which I mean those medical techniques that have to be evaluated by scientific experiment before being accepted as valid) is classed as jing. The studies of biochemistry and pharmacology, because they deal with material chemicals and reactions, are both jing.

The complementary aspect to jing is shen, which is characterized by concepts of the spirit, or thought and consciousness, which are totally non-material. Between these two is an aspect called qi (pronounced 'chi'), which equates to an idea of transformation, or movement, between the two. In China qi is considered a real rather than a theoretical entity, so to call it an idea is not really accurate. However, it is beyond the ability of scientific method to validate, so it has never become familiar to Western practitioners. Rather than trying to define it further, an explanation of what it actually does will be more useful. There are three sources of qi that contribute to its presence in the human body. The first is related to a person's jing characteristics: that which is inherited from the parents, which determines that person's physical constitution - what his or her strong and weak points will be. This is similar to the Western view of genetically determined characteristics, such as inherited diseases like haemophilia and cystic fibrosis. The second type of qi is obtained from the digestion of foods and is therefore dependent on the type of foods eaten and the health of the digestive system. The third type is obtained from the air we breathe and is closely associated with the health of the lungs. The diagnosis that a practitioner of Chinese medicine makes is really an assessment of the condition of a patient's qi in its numerous manifestations. This involves various skills, including an assessment of signs and symptoms (as a Western practitioner would make), checking the qualities and strength of the pulse at the wrist, exerting different pressures (quite different from the way a Western practitioner works), looking at the patient's tongue and observing the general appearance and assessing general points such as the tone of voice and the way a person moves.

In making an assessment of someone's qi, the practitioner will consider various qualities that need to be in balance to achieve a state of good health. If they seem out of balance, that is a key to the cause of the patient's problems and the approach to treating them. The two qualities that the Chinese see as complementary in all aspects of living and non-living matter are called yin and yang. Broadly speaking, the yin aspect of the balance represents the substance or material aspects of a person, while yang is more connected with energy or dynamic processes. As an example of this, think of the relationship between a candle and its flame: the wax and wick represent the yin or substance side of the balance; the flame itself is the yang side.

To Western orthodox medicine, concerned only with aspects of health and disease that can be experimentally validated, there is no concept equivalent to yang, just as there is none for qi or shen. In the jing-qi-shen relationships, jing is the most yin aspect of qi and shen is the most yang aspect. There are other pairs of complementary characteristics that need to be in balance, symbolized by dampness and dryness, heat and cold, outside and inside influences, deficiency and excess, and stagnation and circulation within the body. Beyond these, there are far more divisions of characteristics to be assessed. A practitioner of the Chinese approach will take into account a great deal of information about the patient's constitution during a consultation, whether using acupuncture or herbal medicine as a therapy.

When the picture of where the imbalances occur has been built up, the practitioner will select the appropriate remedy to counteract them. Thus the remedies are classified not because of the chemical constituents they contain (though this may in practice be found to correlate with the Chinese classification) but because of their effects with regard to characteristics such as yin or yang influence, or hot or cold influence, etc. For instance, if there is an excess of 'damp heat' within the body, a remedy that helps to increase the 'dry cold' characteristics would be chosen.

There are five 'tastes' of herbal remedies according to which they are classified. Each taste corresponds to certain characteristic influences that the plants within that group have, as identified by their taste on the tongue. This gives an immediate way of classifying remedies, depending only on the human sense of taste. Of course the taste is a good guide to the type of chemical substances found within a plant; and after observing the effects a group of similar-tasting plants might have, a classification can be made. A similar idea in the West is how people know from experience that hot curries tend to promote a general feeling of warmth and stimulation of the digestion.

The beauty of the Chinese system is that it doesn't rely on any technology, so it was capable of classifying remedies thousands of years before Western scientific medicine was developed. The classifications are as follows.

Pungent-tasting herbs, like the hot spices, are characterized as promoting movement or circulation and are used when there is stagnation. They are employed when 'heat' is deficient and needs to be stimulated. In this respect they are used in a similar way to the 'hot' remedies, notably cayenne, so favoured by the North American physiomedical practitioners for getting rid of 'cold obstructions' in the body. (The convergence of ideas in this respect between these two systems, originating in totally different parts of the world, seems remarkable to me. It shows that in cultures with the minimum of technical support, human ingenuity came up with workable systems of health care that, although unrefined by modern analytical standards, managed to save lives and restore health in the most adverse circumstances.) Pungent remedies are all immediately recognizable by their hot, acrid taste, though there are one or two, such as peppermint, that are classed as pungent and yet have a cooling effect (due to the local anaesthetic properties of menthol). They are contra-indicated in diseases that are characterized by an excess of 'movement' or 'circulation'.

Sweet remedies, such as liquorice (whose botanical name, translated, means 'sugar root'), are considered to have a less extreme effect than the pungent ones and are therefore classed as warming rather than heating. This has an interesting counterpart in Western science, as we know that the body 'burns' sugars to produce energy. These herbs are considered nutritional and 'tonifying', but too much of them can have a harmful cloying effect; hence they should be used with care in conditions where there is an excess of damp or mucus, as they may aggravate this tendency.

Salty-tasting remedies are associated with a cooling influence. Their taste indicates the presence of a high mineral concentration. Examples are the numerous seaweeds known as medicines and foods in the East - in Britain the equivalent would be kelp. In the Chinese system salty remedies are thought to help induce softening and moistening of the tissues, and so are used when the diagnosis suggests an excess of dryness. They are also chosen to treat hard swellings. Appropriately, kelp is the most successful remedy in the treatment of some types of goitre (thyroid gland enlargement) when this is due to an iodine deficiency.

Bitter herbs are classed as having a more extreme action and are called 'cold'. They are a well-known category of remedies in both Chinese and

Western herbal medicine. We know that a bitter taste, by stimulating receptors in the taste-buds, causes a reflex increase in stomach and liver activity, and this has been used to help improve a sluggish digestion. It also seems to be the case that when the digestion is working smoothly, other functions benefit too and a person's sense of wellbeing returns. For this reason the bitters have come to be regarded as general tonics to help in convalescence, etc. They may well have an antifever action, as suggested by their Chinese classification (stimulating the digestion is thought to be one way that a fever can be alleviated).

Sour remedies comprise the fifth classification. They are not associated with either a warming or a cooling action and are neutral in this respect. The taste is that of fruits such as lemons, or very strong tea, and is connected with astringent effects. These remedies are used to reduce abnormal discharges; Western herbal medicine would also choose tannin-containing remedies (tea contains a good deal of tannins) to do the same. Beyond this basic classification, the character of each remedy is further specified to fit it to the character of the illness for which it will be an effective treatment. For instance, there are classes of remedies described as 'tonifying yin and yang', some that tonify only yang, some that 'expel external wind', some that 'clear damp heat' - and many others. As well as individual remedies, there are traditional combinations that are thought to work particularly well together to achieve these effects (just as there are in Western herbal medicine - only we might explain the combination of actions in a different way). They are considered so important that learning them is a much-emphasized part of the training - far more so than it is for Western herbalists. We don't have anything like the same number of set formulations to learn, as most of the 'classic' Western combinations involve two or three herbs at the most.

The advantage of the set combinations is that they can be used by ordinary people who don't have a great deal of medical knowledge. They are easily available at chemist shops in China and are used for minor domestic illnesses that do not require a visit to the doctor. For instance, two called Gan Mao Ling and Gan Mao Qing Re are classified as 'expelling external wind' and are taken to treat 'flu. The names are not the names of the herbs in the combination, but a description of the actions they have. This gives people the information required to buy what will help them, without needing to know the herbs individually. Other popular remedies include those for digestive problems (in the category of 'harmonizing the middle') and coughs (under 'resolving tan'). One combination used externally and internally to promote the healing of wounds is called Yun Nan Bai Yao, which simply means 'the herbs that grow in Yun Nan'. This identifies them quite adequately.

Some herbal remedies are used in both Chinese and Western traditions. Liquorice, ginger, cinnamon, coltsfoot, myrrh and cornsilk all have a traditional name in Chinese characters. Many more herbs used in China are local species that are closely related to medicinally used European species from the same genus. For instance, *Angelica archangelica* is used in Europe, while *Angelica sinensis* (Chinese name, Dang gui) is used in China.

Practitioners in the UK who have qualifications in Chinese herbal medicine are entitled to representation on the Register of Chinese Herbal Medicine. This organization is growing steadily; at present it has about 250 members. The membership is composed mainly of British practitioners of acupuncture who are extending their range of therapies, but some Western-trained herbalists are also choosing to use the Chinese approach. Some members of the

Register are Chinese practitioners who have learnt their skills under the traditional apprenticeship system: if they are deemed to have reached the required standard they are able to join the Register. Until recently Chinese communities in the UK generally had little contact with British culture; this held true for practitioners of their traditional medicine as much as for anyone else. There is now a greater degree of communication, however. As a result, Chinese practitioners have more contact with colleagues who have trained in the West.

A patient who consults a practitioner who is a member of the Register of Chinese Herbal Medicine can have confidence that the practitioner is competent in skills, uses reputable medicines at the correct dosage and adheres to the required standards of safe practice. Consultations will probably include advice about how to maintain a healthy way of life, similar to the approach of a Western herbalist.

The types of problems that Chinese herbal medicine helps are broadly similar to those that Western herbal medicine deals with. The long-term problems that require individual assessment, like skin disease, catarrhal, gynaecological and anxiety/stress problems, can respond well.

The way the remedies are given may be different – most Chinese herbs are prescribed in the form of powders, to be made into teas by the patient. The dosage can be as much as a cupful up to three times a day. The larger doses used and the fact that the remedies have to be imported from the Far East, may mean that the treatments are somewhat costlier than their European equivalents.

USEFUL ADDRESSES

PROFESSIONAL BODIES

National Institute of Medical Herbalists (NIMH)
56 Longbrook Street
Exeter EX4 6AH
Tel. 01392 426022
Send a large stamped addressed envelope for further information and a national list of members. The Institute also runs a BSc degree in herbal medicine at Middlesex University, lasting three years. A fourth year consisting of clinical training entitles students to membership of the NIMH

General Council and Register of Consultant Herbalists (GCRCH)
18 Sussex Square
Brighton
East Sussex BN2 5AA
Tel. 01243 267126
The Council runs a part-time training course, three years long, leading to membership of the GCRCH. Send £1.50 (at the time of going to press) for a prospectus

Register of Chinese Herbal Medicine
4 Glenleigh Terrace
Maidstone Road
Nettlestead
Maidstone
Kent NE18 5EP
Send a stamped addressed envelope and £1.50 (at the time of going to press) for a list of members

OTHER TRAINING COURSES

School of Phytotherapy
Bucksteep Manor
Bodle Street Green
Nr. Hailsham
East Sussex BN27 4RJ
Tel. 01323 833814
Runs full and part-time courses, of four years' duration, training students to the standard required to attain membership of the NIMH

School of Chinese Herbal Medicine
Midsummer Cottage Clinic
Nether Westcote
Kingham
Oxfordshire OX7 6XD
Tel. 01993 830419

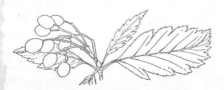

College of Herbs
25 Curzon Street
Basford
Newcastle under Lyme
Staffordshire ST5 0PD
Tel. 01782 711592

HERBAL SUPPLIERS

Suneye Herbs
3 George Street
Balsall Heath
Birmingham B12 9RG
Sells small quantities to the public via
mail-order; send a stamped addressed
envelope for a free price list

The Herbal Apothecary
103 High Street
Syston
Leicester LE7 1GQ
Tel. 0116 2602690
Trade only - minimum order is for ½kg
of dried herbs

CHINESE HERBAL SUPPLIERS

May Way UK Ltd
43 Waterside Trading Estate
Trumpers Way
Hanwell
London W7 2QD
Tel. 0181 893 6873
Trade only, but can supply prescription
requirements for individuals

CHARITIES

**NIMH Ltd Education Fund
Herbal Research (Phytotherapy)**

These registered charities support a range
of projects, including several training
clinics where patients are entitled to
treatment at reduced fees and students
receive clinical training. Research projects
include the setting up of a valuable
database on herbal medicine that is used
by herbal practitioners, orthodox
practitioners and other organizations.

For more information send a stamped
addressed envelope to:

The Fund-Raising Coordinator
PO Box 3
Winchester SO22 8AA

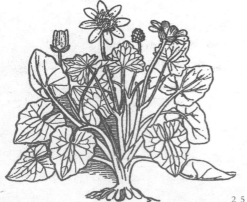